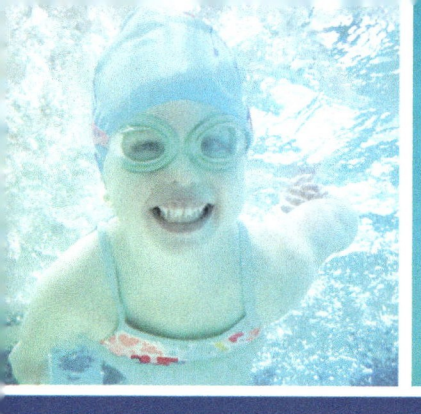

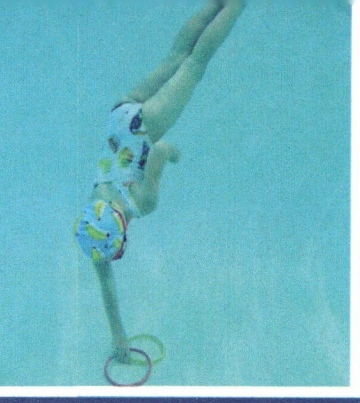

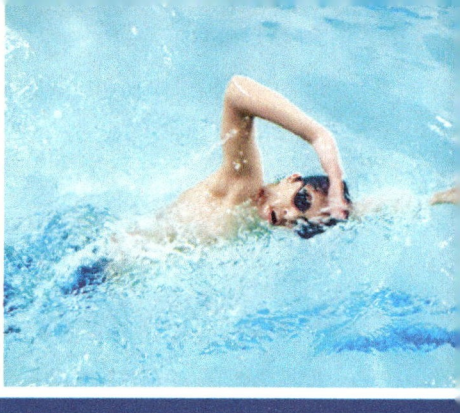

LIFESTYLE SWIMMING INSTRUCTION

The Ultimate Guide to Overcome Fear, Swim Efficiently, and Improve Technique to Become a Better Competitive Swimmer

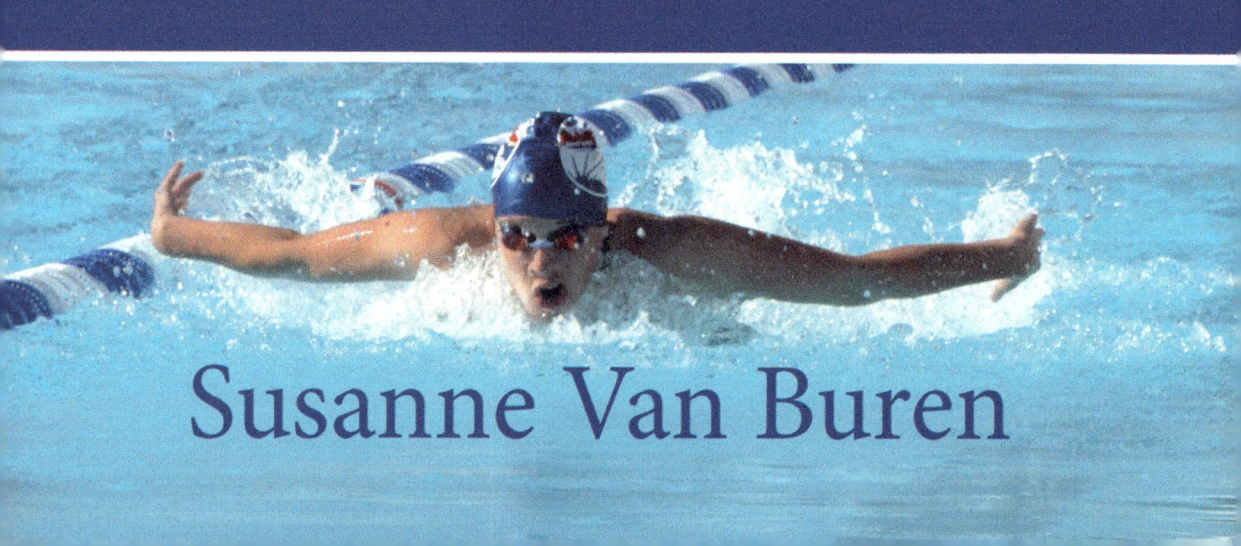

Susanne Van Buren

Lifestyle Swimming Instruction
The Ultimate Guide to Lifestyle Swimming Instruction for Non-Swimmers to Competitive Athletes
Susanne Van Buren © 2021

All rights reserved. Use of any part of this publication, whether reproduced, transmitted in any form or by any means, electronic, mechanical, photocopying, recording, or otherwise, or stored in a retrieval system, without the prior consent of the publisher, is an infringement of copyright law and is forbidden.

While the publisher and author have used their best efforts in preparing this book, they make no representations or warranties with respect to the accuracy or completeness of this book and specifically disclaim any implied warranties of merchantability or fitness for a particular purpose. No warranty may be created or extended by sales representatives or written sales materials. The advice and strategies contained herein may not be suitable for your situation. Neither the publisher nor the author shall be liable for any loss of profit or any other commercial damages, including but not limited to special, incidental, consequential, or other damages. The stories and interviews in this book are true although the names and identifiable information may have been changed to maintain confidentiality.

The publisher and author shall have neither liability nor responsibility to any person or entity with respect to loss, damage, or injury caused or alleged to be caused directly or indirectly by the information contained in this book.

Print ISBN: 978-1-7372587-0-4

Interior and Cover Design by: Fusion Creative Works, FusionCW.com
Book Production by: Aloha Publishing, AlohaPublishing.com
Lead Editor: Heather Goetter

For more information, visit LSIswim.com

Published by Lifestyle Swimming Instruction

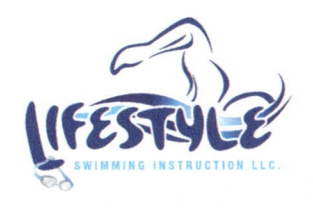

Printed in the United States of America

DEDICATION

To all of you who have inspired me to share my lifelong love of swimming with others. I am so glad we can be on this magical journey together!

CONTENTS

Introduction		11
My Story		15
1.	Why the Lifestyle Swimming Instruction Way?	19
2.	LSI Baby Beginnings	23
3.	LSI Skills #1	29
4.	LSI Skills #2	35
5.	LSI Skills #3	41
6.	LSI Skills #4	47
7.	LSI Clinics: Swim Team Prep	55
8.	LSI Clinics: Adult Beginners	61
9.	LSI Clinics: Adult Intermediate and Advanced	69
Conclusion		77
About Lifestyle Swimming Instruction		79
Acknowledgments		81
About the Author		85
Connect With LSI		87

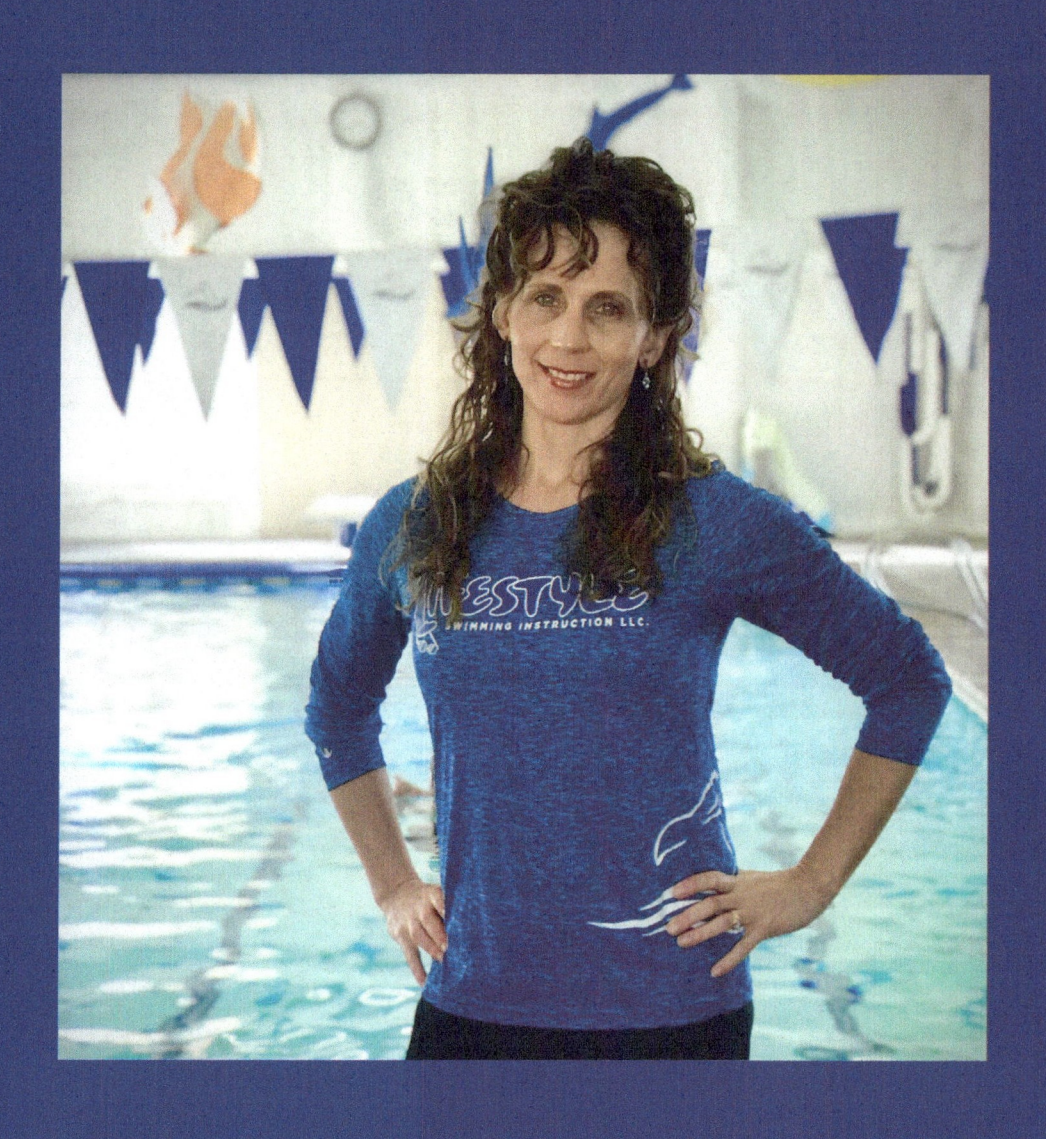

Step out of your comfort zone, take a leap of faith, learn from your mistakes, believe in yourself, and don't forget to record all the miracles you witness along the way!

—Susanne Van Buren

NOTES

INTRODUCTION

Do you really know how to swim?

Is knowing how to swim just getting across the pool in any way, shape, or form? If you asked me 26 years ago, I would not have known how to answer that question. Things have changed drastically in my swimming world since then.

Can everyone learn how to swim? The answer is yes, however, most people think of swimming as *just* getting across the pool. If you use all your energy to get across the pool, swimming with your head up and pounding the water by running your legs and windmilling your arms, you might get to the wall, but that's not really swimming.

What is swimming?

Swimming is peaceful. I know that many people may not think so, but if you do it right, there is no chaos or craziness to it.

Swimming is not like any other sport. It is the only full-body workout, and it requires you to learn how to breathe correctly first before doing any movements.

Lastly, swimming utilizes the properties of the water to move your body through it in the most direct and effortless way.

If you are a teenager or an adult and you decided to take a swim class only to find out your instructor didn't really know how to teach you, then you are *not* alone. Teaching swimming is not for everyone. You either have to know how to teach or be taught how to teach. Even many competitive swimmers have a hard time teaching—since swimming was taught to them at such an early age, they do not remember how they learned. Their mindset might be to teach how to swim fast and get across the pool, but they don't know how to teach the proper technique or mindset from the beginning.

Whatever difficulty you're having with swim lessons, I have been in your shoes: As a teenager embarrassed to be in a class that I knew I wasn't a fit for. As an adult with instructors telling me they didn't know how to teach me how to swim. As a parent watching my little ones in a swim class and asking myself, "Are they really learning or am I just wasting my time and money?"

After many years of struggling with the need and desire for an excellent swim instructor but finding no one who really understood everything about swimming, I began to read swim books, took classes, and never stopped swim lessons for my own children while raising them. I became quite the observer during these years and started teaching swimming myself before I knew all about it. Now my children are so thankful we became a swim family.

During these years of raising my children, I saw so many bad methods of swimming and coaching and read so many books that I became intrigued with learning and teaching the correct methods and the reasons behind them. All three of my children became competitive swimmers. They taught with me as they grew up while racing and occasionally still teach in their adult lives.

I went from thinking I was going to be an elementary education teacher to teaching swimming. It was a long road of trial and error, since in my swimming journey I was taught things I knew were wrong after I tried them. I decided to make my own lesson plans and teach swimming in a whole new way.

I believe that if you teach something right from the beginning, bad habits will not form. Education has always been ingrained in me. Because my mom was my kindergarten teacher, there was no shortage of learning at an early age. In fact, there was always that instilled mindset that you are never too old to learn new tricks!

This LSI method of teaching is to break down strokes similarly to the way that phonics does when you learn to read. Each child needs to understand the

INTRODUCTION

sounds of letters before reading words, just like each person needs to understand each movement their body should make before learning a stroke.

Strokes should not be taught in the beginning with arms and legs. Rather, they must be broken down. First and foremost, how do you go under the water correctly without getting water up your nose? Learning to swim should not happen on a swim team. Students should know all four competitive swim strokes well—Freestyle, Backstroke, Breaststroke, and Butterfly—before entering a swim team. Students should understand all technicalities of each stroke before they hear the words, "It's time to race!"

So you ask, "Why am I hearing this now? My child learned on a swim team and now has injuries and bad technique." The dictionary definition of swimming is: *The sport or activity of propelling oneself through water using the limbs.* That is the definition of doggie paddling, which is why swimming is often taught incorrectly. I have seen it almost every day for the last 20 years since I started teaching. When a new client says that their child knows how to swim, the chances are very high that the child is either doggie paddling or close to it.

By learning each of the LSI skills, you will understand the importance of the LSI definition of swimming:

*Swimming is a sport like no other, also known as the most technical sport and lifesaving skill there is. It's all about the understanding of your body being in the most relaxed state of mind and learning the correct muscle memory; making proper bubbles when submerging your body in water; the forward movement of your whole body to become more fluid in the water by the natural engagement of your core and the rotation of your hips that require different movements in each stroke; kicking from your hips and **not** your knees; the proper placement of the hands; and balancing your body with your head in line with your spine. Your body eventually becomes one with the water with each possible movement.*

I have now been teaching swimming for over 20 years. My small one-woman operation has turned into a thriving, multi-level, multi-instructor business. I hope to change the swimming definition permanently, so people understand the importance of truly swimming and not just moving their limbs to get across the pool.

These are LSI's goals:

- To teach all ages, from babies to adults, in order to eliminate drownings by teaching safety first.

- To train people to teach swimming with proper form in order to reduce swimmers' injuries and stop wasting years with bad muscle memory.

- To have everyone understand the water and learn how to feel it rather than fight it, by becoming one with the water.

Everyone can learn how to swim correctly at any age.

No matter what you do, never give up, and do not let your children give up. Swimming is the most important sport and lifesaving skill there is. Everyone should know how to swim; it's a better life to live!

MY STORY

The family I grew up in was not a "water family." However, when we visited relatives, we'd always look for hotels that had a pool. As the youngest, I was terrified of water. My siblings seemed to enjoy it a lot more than I did. In fact, one time my 21-year-old brother thought I would get over my fear if he threw me into one of the hotel pools. I was 14 years old at the time. Guess what happened? I sank straight to the bottom. He quickly jumped in after me and dragged me to the surface. Luckily the pool was no more than 6 feet, so he could reach me pretty easily. After that I was even more scared.

My family's usual vacation spot was beautiful Panama City, Florida. When I was a toddler, I would crawl up my mom's leg, screaming, anytime she brought me close to the waves. She felt my pain because she was a non-swimmer and had a fear of the water as well. We would go to the beach frequently and I always chose to make sandcastles instead of playing in the water. As I got a little older, my friends would invite me to pool parties. I would either make excuses not to go or spend the time clinging to the sides of the pool for dear life.

At 16 years old, I decided to take a swim class. To my horror, my swim instructor was a cute guy in a speedo, and I was placed in a class with kids much younger than me. He had no idea what to do with me and couldn't understand why I just didn't get it. I lasted only a few lessons.

In college, I decided to give swim lessons another try. Their approach was to have everyone wear life jackets. How do you learn how to swim in a lifejacket?

LIFESTYLE SWIMMING INSTRUCTION

I lasted a few months. I took another class later at another college and the instructor was pregnant. I didn't learn much because I was distracted and concerned about her baby every time she dove in the water. Between that and the terrified feeling I experienced every time I was required to go in the deep end, I ended that class still dealing with fear and with no understanding of the water.

Fast-forward a few years. I had gained 51 pounds by the time I delivered my first child. I was not happy with myself. It was an awful feeling not being able to bend over and tie my own shoes. My neighbor persuaded me to try water aerobics at a friend's house. I was desperate. The whole time I was either glued to the pool wall or clutching the pool noodle like my life depended on it. I was known as the one who couldn't tread water. However, I kept going and eventually learned to love it. I lost all my extra weight within six months.

Through the next two pregnancies, I kept up with water aerobics and other forms of exercise. I didn't gain as much weight, but more importantly, I stayed consistent in the water. I regularly enrolled in Mommy and Me Water Baby classes. My oldest child would scream in the water like I did as a baby, but I persisted. It was embarrassing, but I forced us to stick with it as much as possible. I didn't want this inherited behavior to continue.

When my kids were a little older, I decided to take adult swimming classes again. I actually started enjoying the water more once I learned how to blow bubbles, dive for rings, and do deep bobs. This was a game changer for me. Water became intriguing.

As I learned, so did my kids. I noticed that every time I took them to a new swim instructor, they were taught totally different things. One instructor would work on how to blow bubbles, the next would concentrate on form, and another would emphasize floating. I took mental notes all the time because it was clear that there was no concrete method to learn to swim and understand the water.

When my oldest started school, I decided to work hard and get this swimming thing down. I took a fun adult class and met new friends who were at my level but had their own stories. Once I started to swim laps, the instructor

MY STORY

encouraged me to teach. I decided to go for it, *not* because I wanted to teach, but because my membership would be cheaper if I did!

I became a swim instructor when my kids were between 2-5 years old, before I really knew about the water, before I knew how to swim well or do laps well, and before I was even confident in the deep end.

Something clicked for me one day when I was teaching an adult class. An older lady shared her traumatic water story during a lesson. There were many adults in the class dealing with fear, but I had other students who were ready to take off doing laps. They were all at different levels with backgrounds ranging from paralyzing fear to no fear at all. Some were survival swimmers who moved their legs and arms in the water very inefficiently. I told the aquatic director that I needed these adults in three different class levels in order to teach them correctly. The director told me, "Oh, all adults know how to swim!"

It was clear to me by then that I wasn't the only one who struggled with growing up a non-swimmer. Most people think they know how to swim. Most people don't understand how you can grow up near beaches, pools, rivers, and lakes without learning to swim. However, there are plenty of adults who don't know how to swim.

Swimming isn't just getting yourself from point A to point B as fast as possible. It involves so much more. Safety, breathing, floating, and form are just a few of the tools involved in swimming and most people have never been taught any of those things correctly.

Soon after I started teaching swimming, I joined a master's swim class. A friend of mine joined me and both she and I started getting into the nuances of swimming well. I was hooked. I started swimming every day, and when I wasn't swimming, I was thinking about swimming—my form, how to flip turn, the best hand positions. The more I practiced, the more endurance I had. The more endurance I had, the better I swam. My confidence in all depths of water skyrocketed.

After a few years, I got an offer to help coach a high school swim team. That took me to the next level. I learned so much about every stroke. I learned what works and what doesn't work. I also learned it can be great to teach older children, especially if they are committed to learn and get better. That was a good year for Boise's Capital High School! We had the best team.

I ended up taking more and more classes of drills and would practice them on my own. I discovered things I hadn't ever been taught. It was crazy to me. I figured out the only way the water can hold you is if you relax. No one had ever taught me that in any of my lessons or practices. During that time, I actually learned how *not* to swim and just relax in the water.

Then my children became competitive swimmers. That was a whole new world. It was fun to watch them work so hard at something and succeed. It encouraged me to swim more. I ended up teaching so many classes that I had to start teaching privately just to fit it into my schedule. That was when Lifestyle Swimming Instruction, LLC, was born.

Swimming isn't just a sport; it's a necessity!

> I will be forever grateful to the nurse who got me through my very first birth. I had no idea what I was doing, and this amazing woman taught my husband and I how to time each contraction, how to relax through the hardest part, and how to trust the doctors and nurses. It was a life-changing method and so helpful that not only did I use it for my two other births, but I integrated it into other aspects of my life: know what's coming, relax and don't freak out, breathe, trust the experts, relax, do it all again.
>
> I use a method of coaching that teaches consistency and timing. My story makes it clear that swimming is more than its dictionary definition. I wanted to be like that one nurse who was unlike all of the others so I could make a difference in the lives of swimmers.

1

WHY THE LIFESTYLE SWIMMING INSTRUCTION WAY?

"The water is your friend—you don't have to fight with water, just share the same spirit as the water, and it will help you move."

—Alexander Popov, Olympic Gold Metalist

Lifestyle Swimming Instruction is unlike any other swimming program.

Swimming should be the first sport we learn. We need to be taught kinetic muscle memory and learn to understand how fluid and graceful our bodies can be in the water. Struggling in the water in any way is not swimming.

At Lifestyle Swimming Instruction, we give students the tools they need to be safe in the water. We give them the confidence they need to succeed both in and out of the water. Approximately one in five people who die from drowning are children 14 years old or younger. For every child who dies from drowning, another five receive emergency care for nonfatal submersion injuries. And the rate of near drowning is much higher, as not all near drownings are reported.

Our children are our investments. People want to have their children learn quickly how to get around the pool so they can enjoy and relax in the sun. Quickly learning the basics of swimming does not teach children to think critically in all water situations, but just to survive to get themselves out of the water. Swimming well takes time and repetition. Swimming cannot be taught in 10-minute classes. Babies who are taught to go under and roll over before they understand their correct bubbles can develop a chemical imbalance if they inhale too much pool water. No one should be forced to go under the water when they are not ready. This instills fear, stress, and extra movements that are unnecessary in a swimming journey.

Let LSI take you and your family through a swim journey. You will learn to love the water and it will help you physically, emotionally, and mentally. Proper swimming brings many positives, including the following:

- Reduction of injuries
- Lower drowning rates
- Increased confidence
- Improved health and fitness
- Proper form and good habits for competition

The Value of the LSI Methods

The most important elements of swimming are safety first, the understanding of the water, breathing correctly, and learning technique the correct way from the beginning. As each stroke is taught and understood, speed can be introduced. If swimming is not taught in this way, injuries will occur.

There is much more to swimming than just propelling yourself using your limbs. Toddlers who are consistent in swim lessons do not have to move their bodies much to get around in the water. They have already learned how to go under correctly, back float, glide, glide on front, roll from front to back, and start the movements of their first stroke, the Elementary Backstroke.

Learning how to swim doesn't just happen on its own. It takes effort and training with the right methods to become a fluid swimmer. However, once you understand how to relax, rotate, and swim laps, you will be extremely confident. The time spent learning these foundational techniques is worth it.

WHY THE LIFESTYLE SWIMMING INSTRUCTION WAY?

At LSI We Focus on These Three Things:

1. Learning Technique:

At LSI, every skill is taught and practiced until mastered. Learning technique before speed is crucial. Learning technique takes time and consistency, but it is well worth the effort to discover the magical feel of how the water works with your body. Proper technique is the foundational building block for great swimming. It doesn't matter if you swim for leisure, on a summer league, a high school team, a college level team, a nationally ranked team, in triathlons, or if you want to become the next Michael Phelps. In order to reach your potential, you must have a solid foundation in proper stroke technique that leads to progression in your desired goal.

2. Building Endurance:

Swimming endurance is important for health, safety, and performing well in competitions. After you have successfully accomplished the proper stroke technique, your next step is to practice while building your endurance. At LSI we teach drills to improve endurance while still focusing on technique. This allows you to really feel the water. It is during this practice that muscle memory is imprinted and reinforced.

3. Increasing Speed:

The third step is swimming fast with excellent technique and holding that technique at a race pace. Speed is the last skill to work on after technique and endurance have been mastered. At this point, the drills and repetition are muscle memory.

The mental training to establish proper technique is where many swimmers and coaches struggle. If coaches only stress going fast and the swimmer's technique is not good, that swimmer will struggle, no matter their age. Often swimmers who have made it to the collegiate level have to be held back because their technique is not where it needs to be in order to compete. That is why LSI teaches the correct body position and the correct technique before teaching endurance and speed.

If you haven't been taught proper technique before, learning how to swim correctly can be a long process. However, once you have a solid stroke foundation, you will start to swim faster, and your time difference will be noticeable especially in longer swimming events. With patience, persistence, and hard work, your swimming will begin to feel magical.

2

LSI BABY BEGINNINGS

Amanda was traveling with her 1-year-old twins by herself. She decided to take them to their motel pool. When it was time to get them out of the water, she sat one of the children on the side of the pool. That little one decided to get up and run away while she was getting the other one. All she could remember from our class at the time was yelling, "Humpty Dumpty!" Humpty Dumpty is LSI's song all parents sing with babies sitting down on the edge of pool. No child is allowed to enter the water until everyone is ready. This teaches all babies to listen and only go into the water on command, teaching them to be safe around the water. Guess what that little girl did after she heard that? Yes, she immediately sat down so her mom was able to get her.

The LSI Baby Beginnings program teaches floating, swimming, and safety with fun songs, toys, and parental involvement. Babies respond well to songs, repetitive movements, and a lot of love. Each skill is taught and practiced for a reason. The skills build on one another as the child gains confidence and proficiency.

Having parents in the water helps the babies get comfortable. It also gives parents fun exercises to do with their babies and good quality time with them. The parents get a workout as well. Each skill is practiced, instilling the children with confidence and muscle memory in the water, getting them prepared for the next class without their parent.

LSI's method does not just teach babies how to survive in the water. It teaches them to understand how the water holds them. They learn how to relax

LIFESTYLE SWIMMING INSTRUCTION

their bodies and not fight the water to get across the pool. They start learning nose bubbles before they go under the water. If babies are not taught this, they can ingest pool water, which can lead to a chemical imbalance.

With LSI's methods, parents are given essential skills to teach their babies the number one rule: Do not enter the water without their parent.

In this class, children learn the rules of the pool, work on muscle memory and good technique with songs and props, and learn how their bodies work in the water. They leave this class with no more fear, enjoying going under and loving the water, and knowing they should never get in the pool without their parent or guardian.

To graduate this class, they will learn how to walk in two feet of water and be comfortable going under and coming up. Some 1-2-year-olds will even know how to float on their backs by themselves.

Baby Beginnings Skills

Skill 1: Nose Bubbles and Hums

Baby Beginners learn how to correctly go underwater by taking a breath above the water with their mouth open first, then zipping their lips and humming like they would to a song or by blowing out their nose. This forms nose bubbles, so they do not inhale any water.

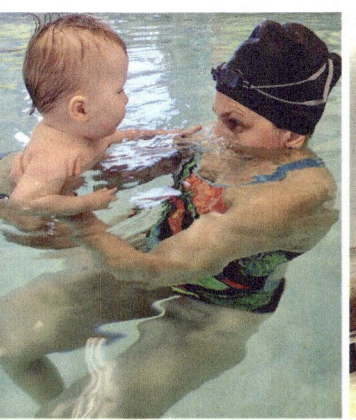

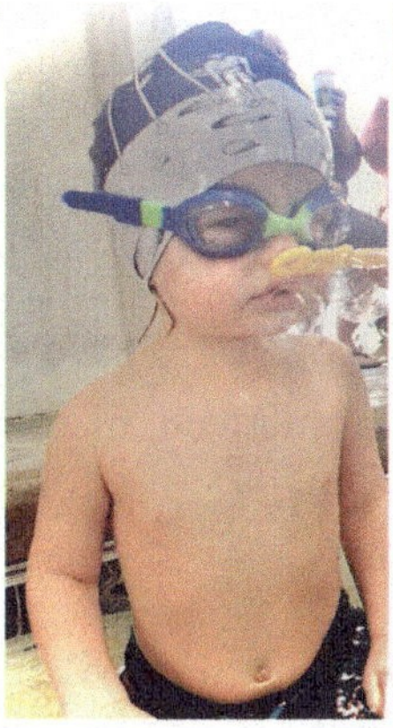

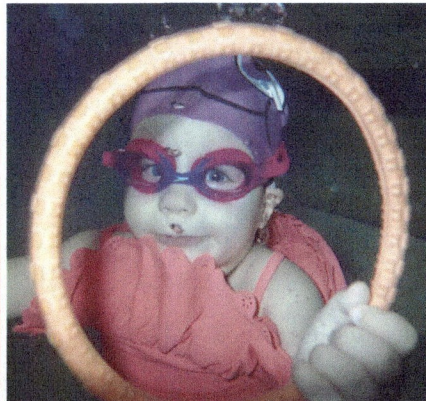

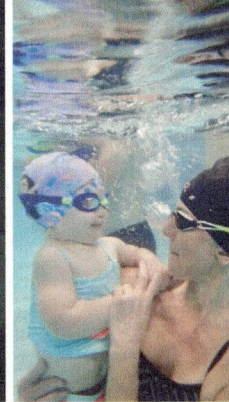

Skill 2: Getting Used to Water Over Their Heads

Many children fear getting water on their faces and being unable to wipe it away. Many babies do not like water over their heads. This skill teaches them to learn to love the water.

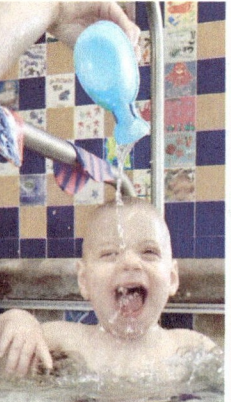

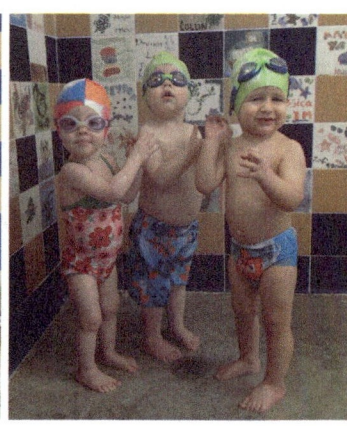

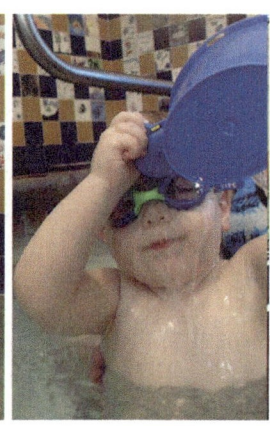

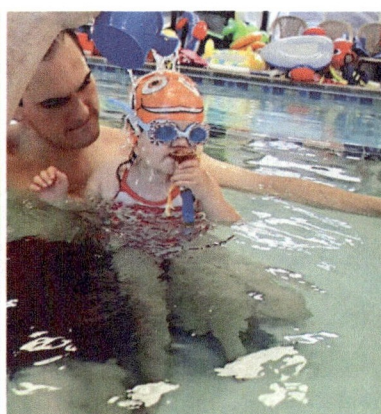

Skill 3: Walking in Shallow Water (Tic-Toc)

Baby Beginners learn how to walk in two feet of water. This teaches control, balance, and confidence. They learn not to run and jump but control their movements to a tic-toc beat. This also teaches them to go under the water and come back up with confidence before they are in a class by themselves.

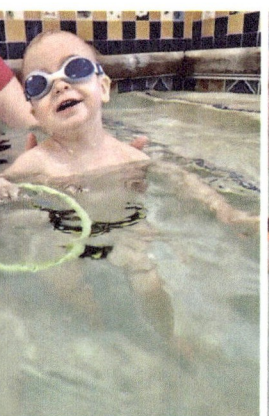

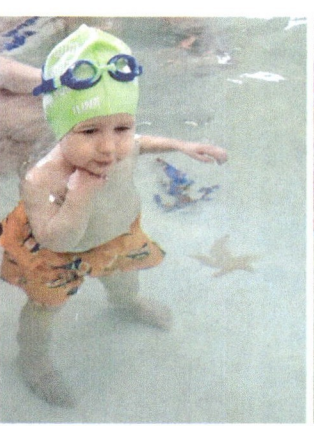

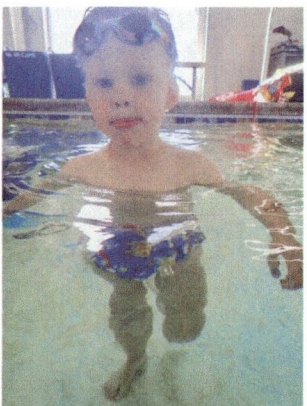

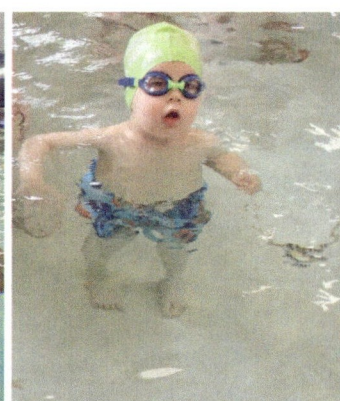

LIFESTYLE SWIMMING INSTRUCTION

Skill 4: Climbing Out (Elbow-Elbow-Knee-Knee)

This skill teaches Baby Beginners the safe way to climb out of a pool and helps them get stronger by pulling themselves out of the water.

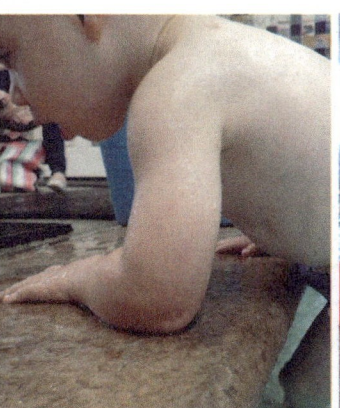

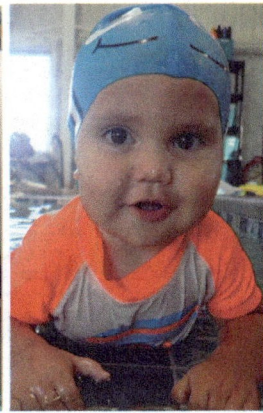

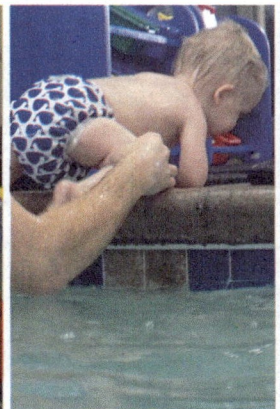

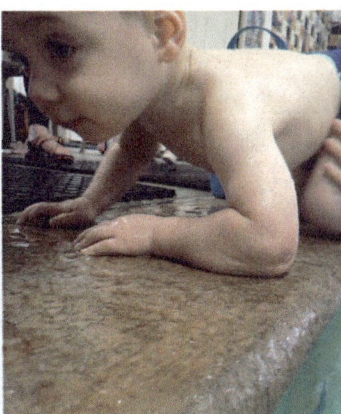

Skill 5: Safety (Humpy-Dumpty and Curl Toes)

Baby Beginners learn not to go in the water before their parent or guardian is already in the water. Babies learn to safely enter a pool from either sitting on the edge or standing with toes curled at the edge. Parents practice teaching their babies how to jump on their command into the water and away from the edge. The babies learn to trust the water, their parent, and the instructor.

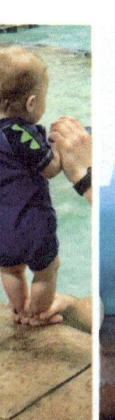

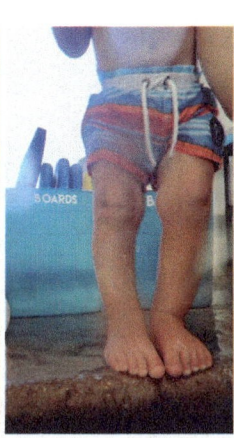

"LIFE LOOKS BETTER UNDERWATER."

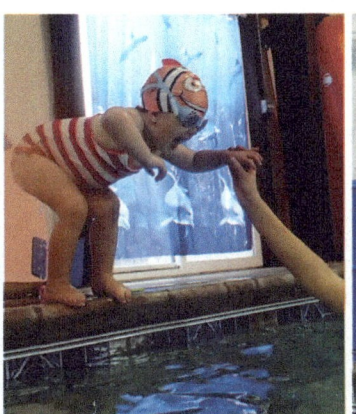

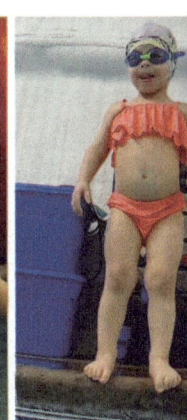

Skill 6: 1, 2, 3, Scoop

Parents scoop the baby in the water, touching their ear to the water on both sides with a one, two, three, hum. This helps the baby get comfortable with the water going right by their ears and face. Once they know how to do nose bubbles, they are scooped under the water sideways.

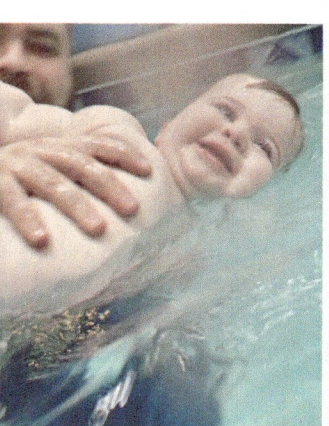

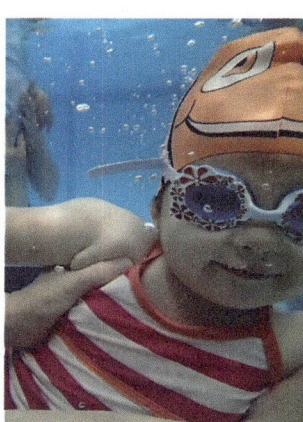

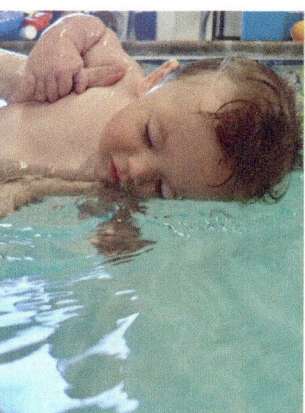

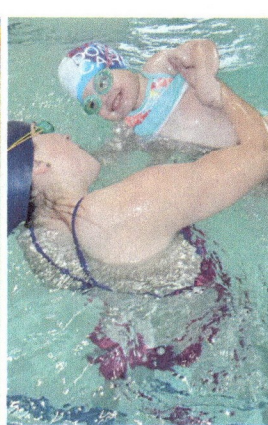

Skill 7: Back Float

Baby Beginners learn how to trust the water to hold them while their parent or instructor assists them in a back float. Some will be able to do this on their own by the time they are 1 to 2 years old.

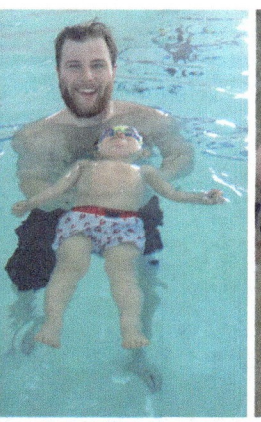

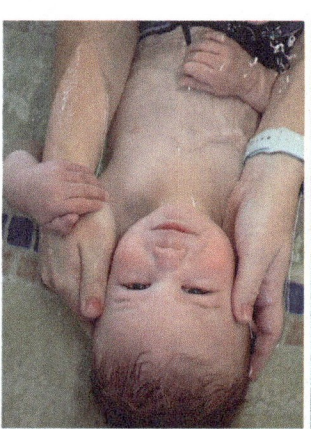

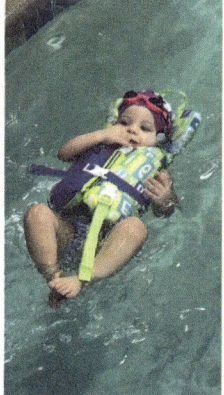

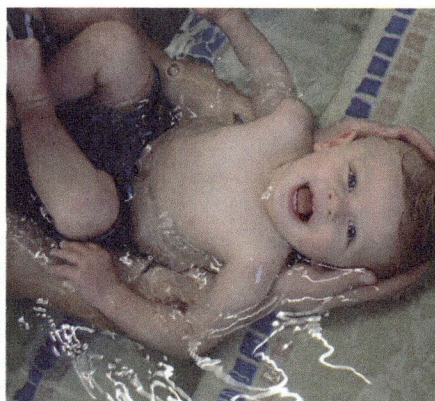

LIFESTYLE SWIMMING INSTRUCTION

Skill 8: Noodle Time

Baby Beginners learn how to balance and move themselves in the water on a noodle to learn to relax their bodies and get used to the feel of moving through the water.

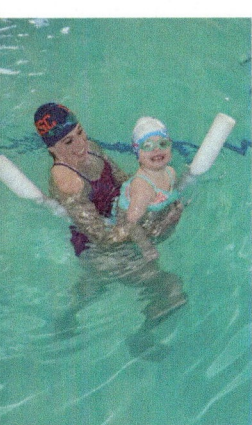

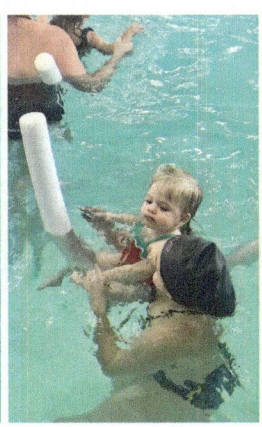

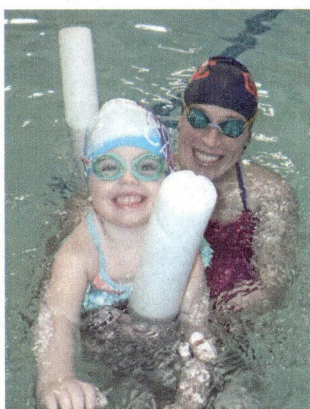

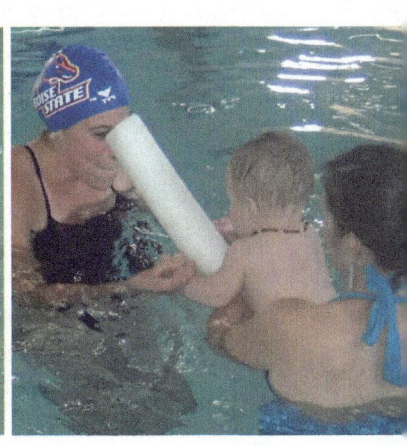

LSI BABY BEGINNINGS PARTING SHOTS

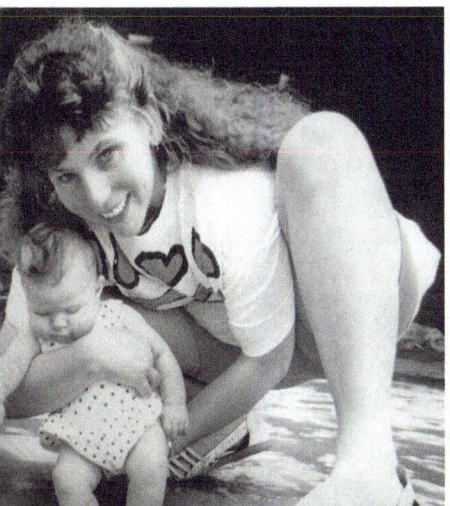

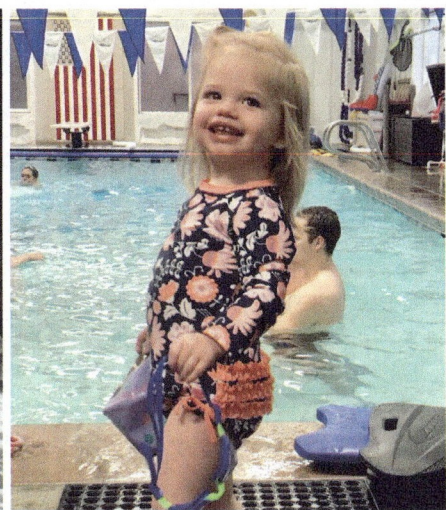

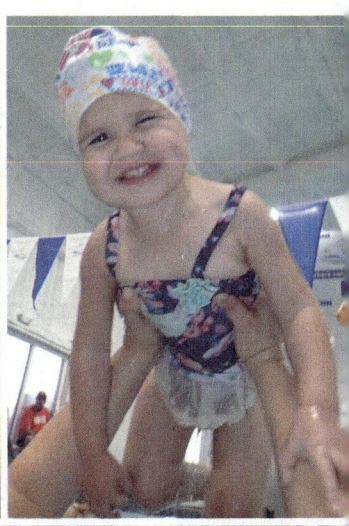

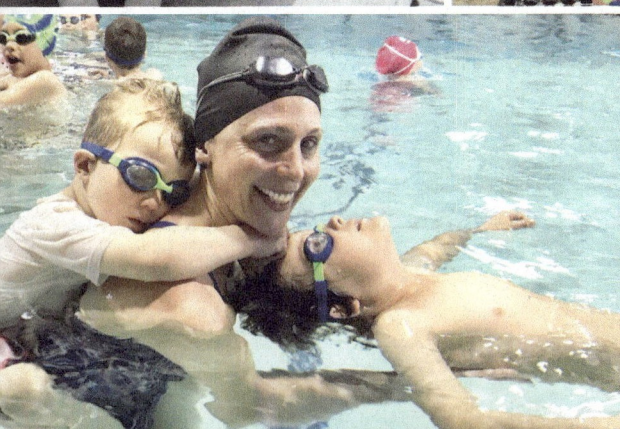

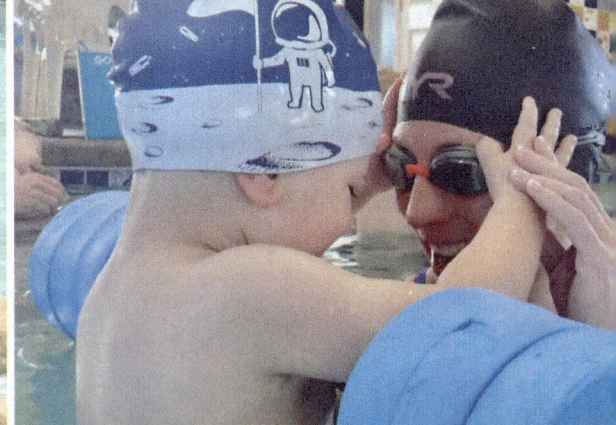

3

LSI SKILLS #1

Shawna, a mom of three children came to LSI looking for a different avenue to learn swimming. She had done some swimming growing up but didn't have confidence in the water. She'd placed her children in swimming lessons elsewhere but had a couple scary experiences with them in water. The most recent was with her youngest child at 3 years of age. The child had been sinking and unresponsive. They had to resuscitate. Shawna and her husband joined LSI's adult program and enrolled all three children in the appropriate levels. She thought her youngest child would not progress right away. However, the 3-year-old listened and understood the pool rules, learned how to let the water hold her by doing back floats, and learned how to go under the water correctly by doing nose bubbles. She even went off the diving board on the second day she was in class. She now loves the water and enters the pool happily every time.

This is the first class students do in a group without their parent or guardian. They will learn how to be in a group setting and listen to pool rules so they never enter the water without permission. They will learn to try skills they might not want to try, but love doing them once they learn. This class is intended to help young children learn safety, go under the water correctly, dive for rings in three to five feet of water, back float, front glide, go from their front to their back, and learn to do the Elementary Backstroke.

LIFESTYLE SWIMMING INSTRUCTION

Pre-Skills:

Students must either graduate from Water Babies or be 3½ years old with the attention span to sit and listen to instruction and be comfortable walking in two feet of water.

Skills #1

Skill 1: Bubbles and Hums

Students learn how to take a breath above the water in through their mouth and out through their nose. This forms nose bubbles under the water so no water goes up their nose and they do not inhale water while going under. Humming to music under the water forms nose bubbles also.

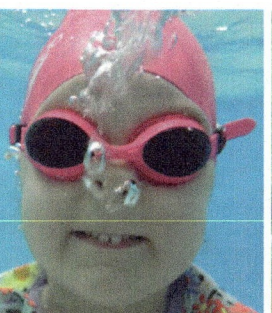

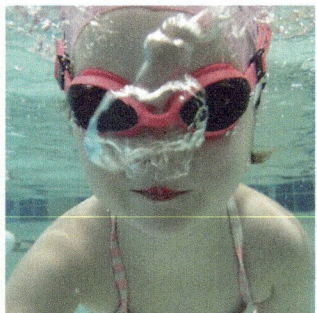

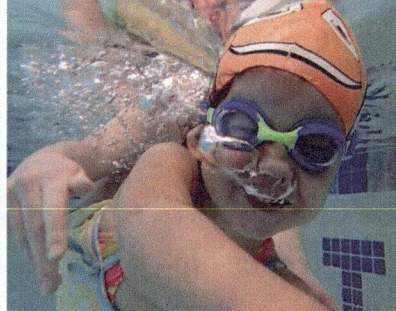

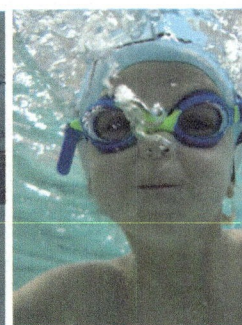

Skill 2: Back Floats

Students learn how to trust the water to hold them by floating on their back.

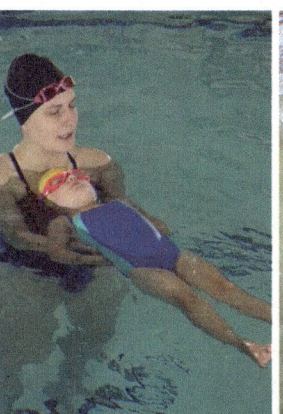

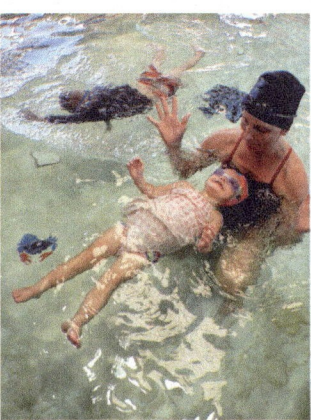

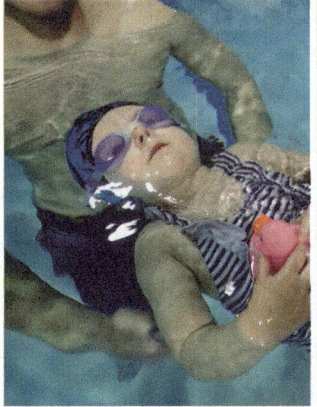

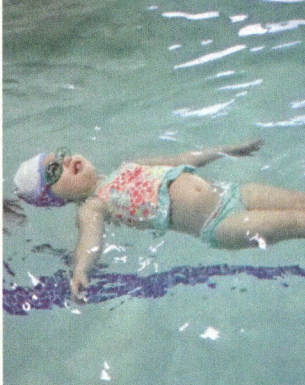

LSI SKILLS #1

Skill 3: Glides

Students learn how the water helps move them when they are relaxed and their head is in-line with their spine, each arm parallel to the other, reaching out as far as they can, touching each ear, and with toes touching.

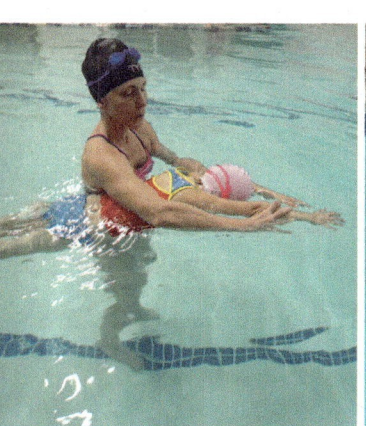

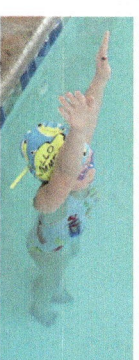

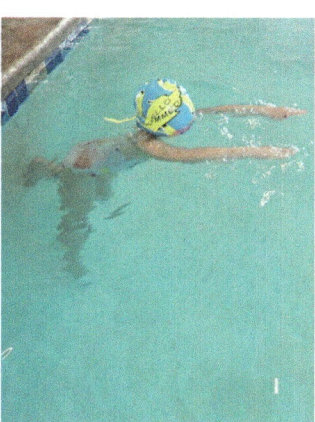

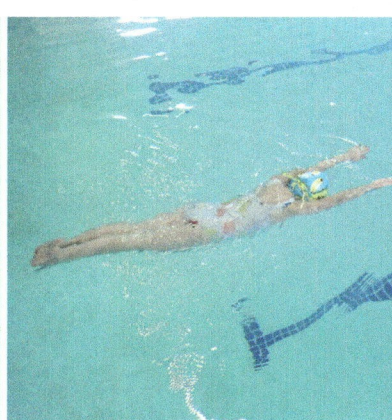

Skill 4: Deep Bobs

Students practice deep water bobs correctly, using their arms to raise and lower their body while legs do the Whip Kick and arms do a jumping jack. This teaches them how they don't have to work hard for the water to hold them.

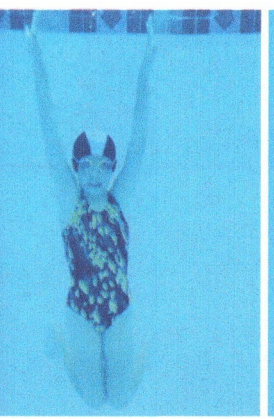

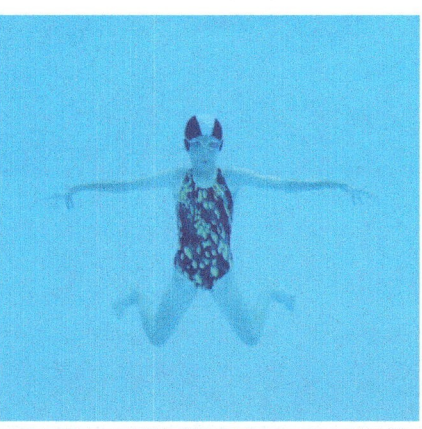

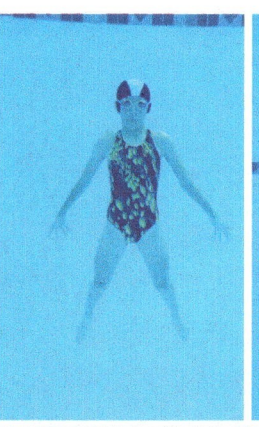

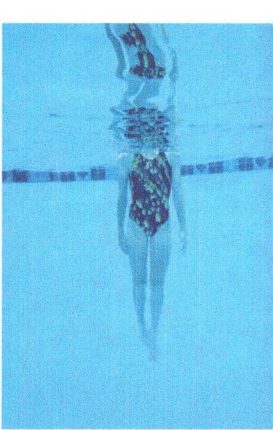

Skill 5: Glide, Reach, Roll

This is the foundational move for many skills. Students will glide for two seconds, keeping their left ear on their left arm, pulling their right arm straight down to their side while rotating their hips and then ending up on their back.

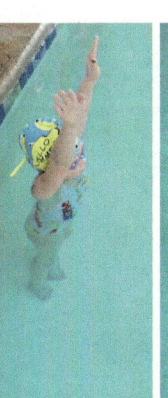

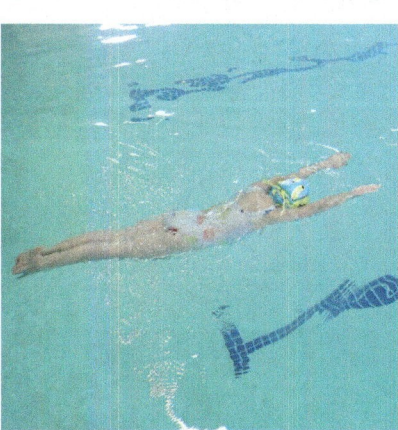

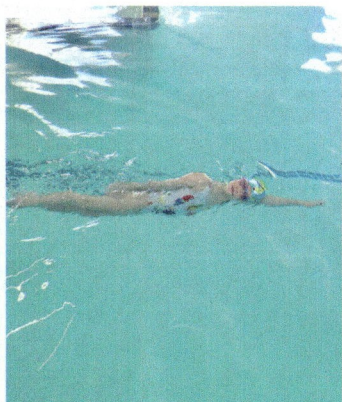

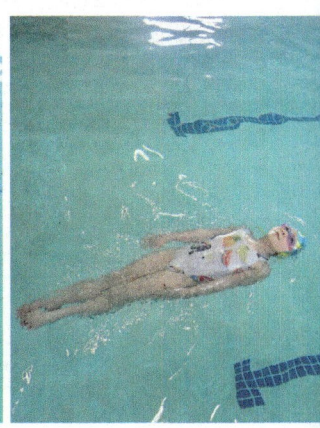

Skill 6: Elementary Backstroke

Starting with a back float, hands slide up each side while the feet go back as far as possible—keeping hips on top of the water. Arms move straight out while feet turn out—keeping knees in line with shoulders. Arms come straight down while pushing with heels, drawing two half circles with toes, ending with toes touching to form a back glide—creating the first kick, the Whip Kick.

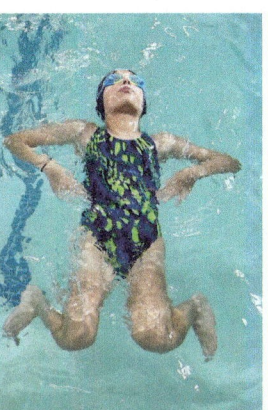

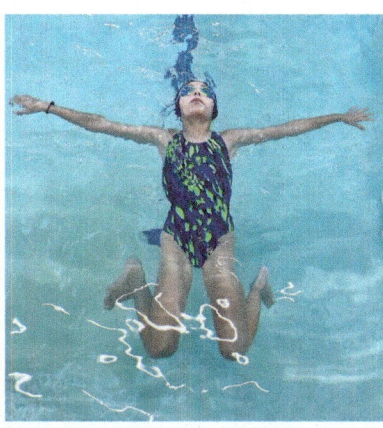

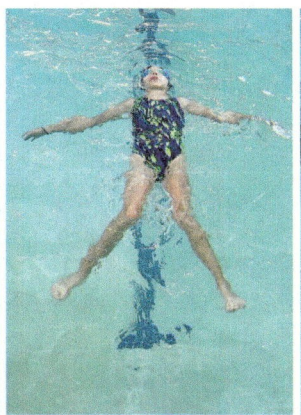

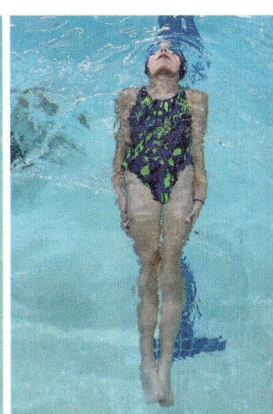

LSI SKILLS #1

Skill 7: Rings (3-5 feet)

Students learn how to go underwater correctly to retrieve an object at the bottom of the pool three to five feet down, initially with help, then eventually by themselves.

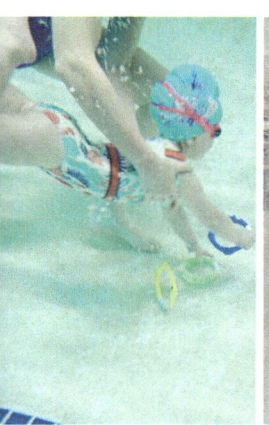

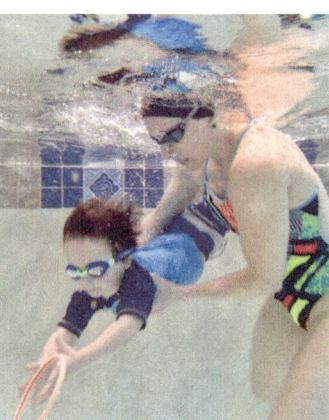

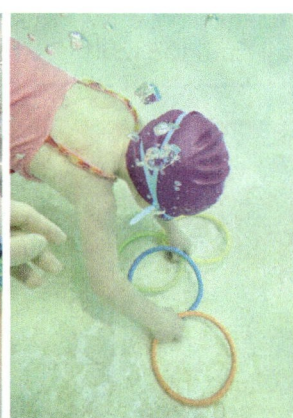

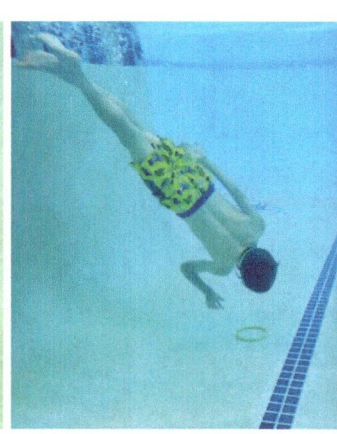

Skill 8: Jumping In (Off Diving Board)

Students learn to jump into the water correctly, overcoming any fear of heights or of jumping in the water.

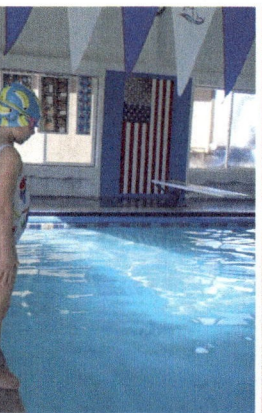

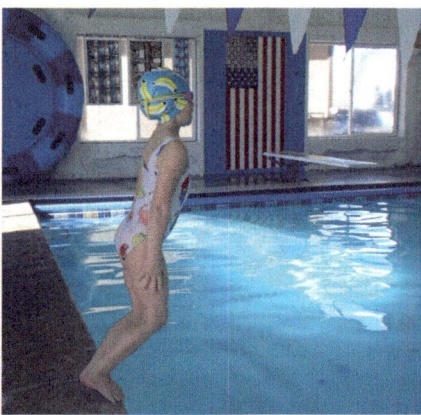

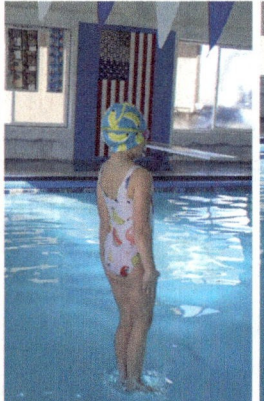

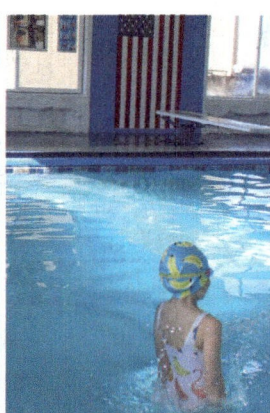

LIFESTYLE SWIMMING INSTRUCTION

> ### Skill 9: Sitting Dives
>
> Students are ready to learn their first taught dive. Students sit on the pool edge with arms reaching up to the ceiling behind their ears, hands pancaked together. They need to bend at their waist, push the wall away with their feet, while keeping their head in line with their spine, and go into a glide once they push away from the wall.

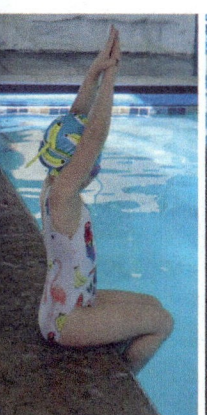

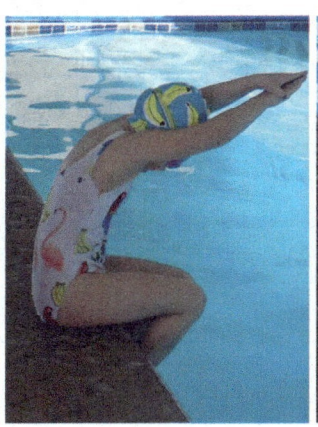

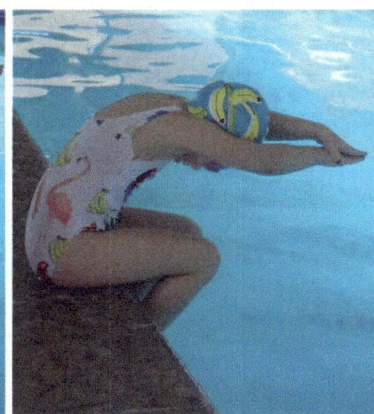

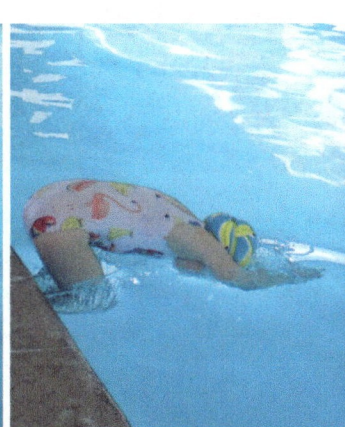

LSI SKILLS #1 PARTING SHOTS

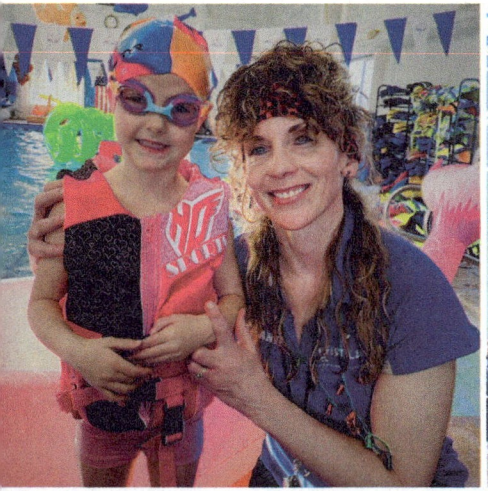

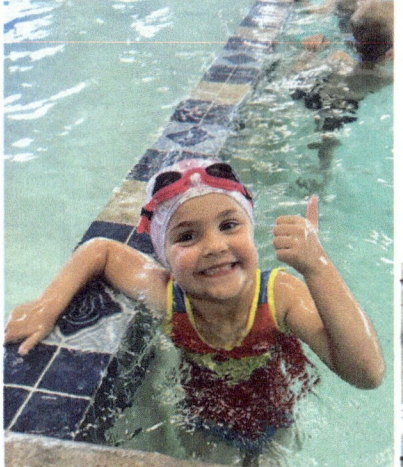

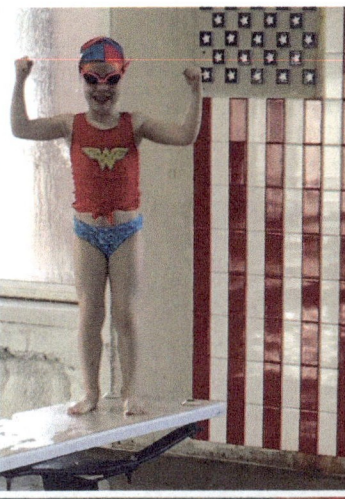

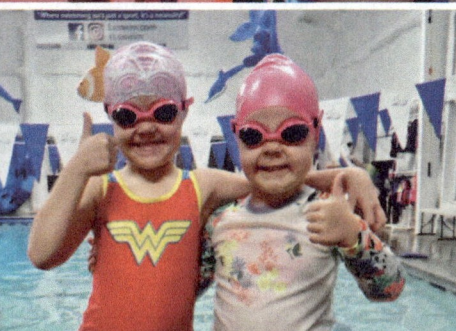

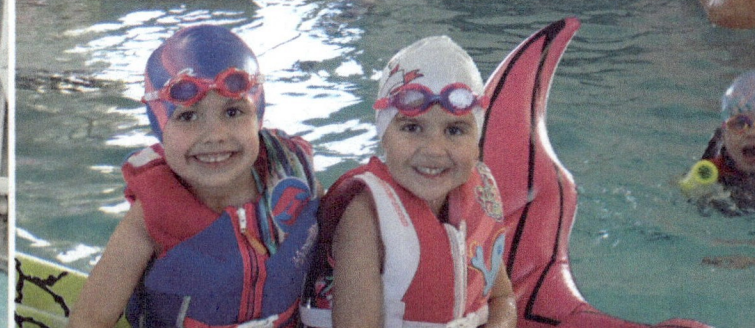

4

LSI SKILLS #2

Yaneth first heard of LSI when she was in search of swim lessons for her 6-year-old son. He had already taken classes elsewhere but had not enjoyed it and expressed no desire to return. She was afraid he would quit swimming altogether and grow up to be an adult non-swimmer. After only the first lesson, her son asked to return for more lessons. She was relieved and impressed at the effect just one day of lessons had on her son. The son had a taste of other swim lessons and was immediately convinced that LSI was the place for him. He continued to thrive with the LSI instructors. They were effective, efficient, consistent, and compassionate.

LSI Skills #2 is the second group class that teaches students how to understand the water and how to move through it with grace, becoming one with the water. The skills students learn in the class are diving for rings by themselves, treading in all depths of water with no help, continuing to perfect their Elementary Backstroke, starting to Flutter Kick, kick on their side, and then form their next stroke—Freestyle. They will start learning to do sitting dives on their own with no help and start standing dives.

Pre-Skills:

Students must either graduate from the LSI Skills #1 or know how to Glide, Reach, and Roll with little help and be comfortable in the deep end with an instructor.

Skills #2

Skill 1: Rings (3-10 feet)

The students learn how to go underwater correctly to retrieve an object or touch the bottom of the pool by themselves. Some may dive down to 10 feet in this class.

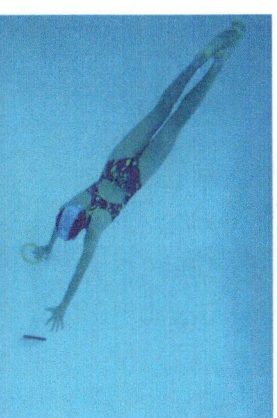

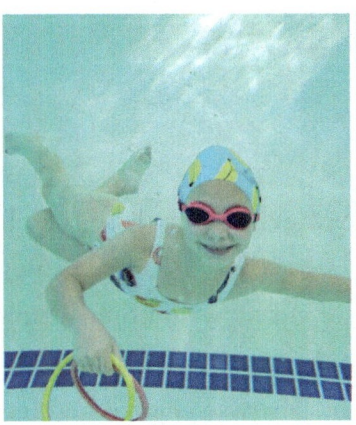

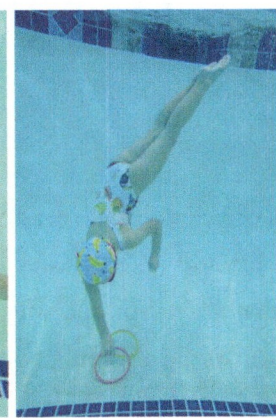

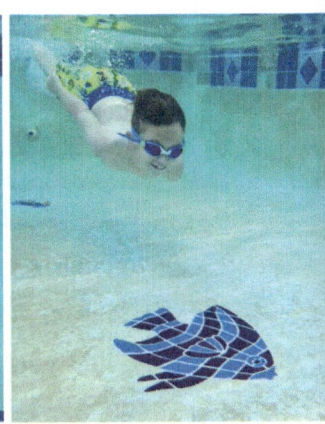

Skill 2: Treading

Students learn to tread water by scooping their arms toward them while doing the Whip Kick they have already been taught in Elementary Backstroke. They will learn to do this with their heads up in 10 feet of water without help once they graduate from this class.

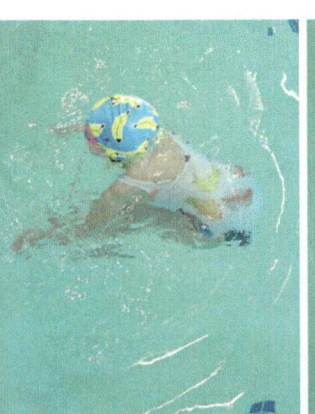

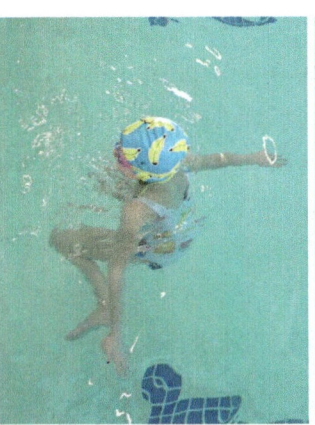

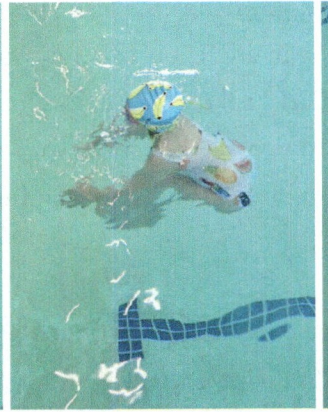

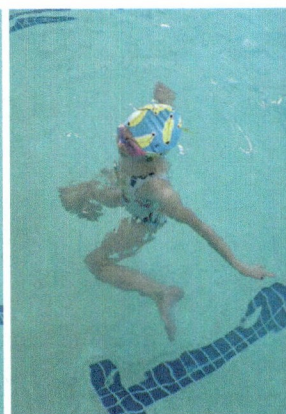

LSI SKILLS #2

Skill 3: Perfecting Elementary Backstroke

Starting with a back float, hands slide up each side while the feet go back as far as possible, keeping hips on top of the water. Arms move straight out while feet turn outward, keeping knees in line with shoulders. Arms come straight down to the side while pushing with heels, drawing two half circles with toes, ending with toes touching, forming a back glide. This creates the first kick, the Whip Kick.

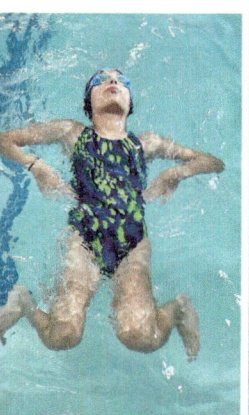

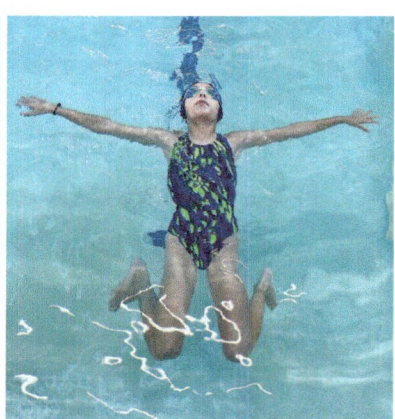

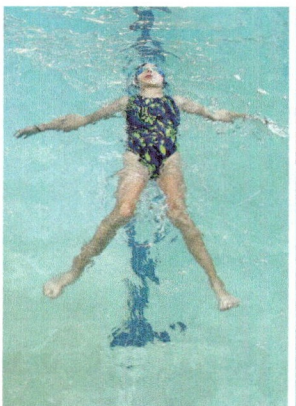

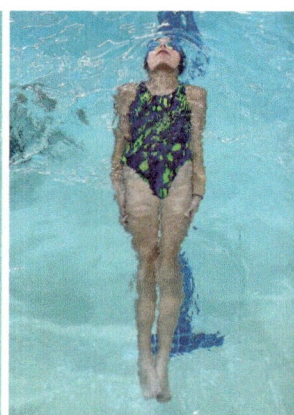

Skill 4: Flutter Kicks

Students learn to kick with proper form, from their hips.

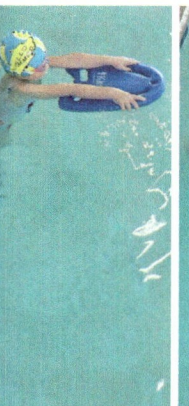

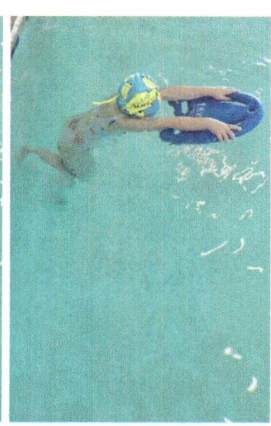

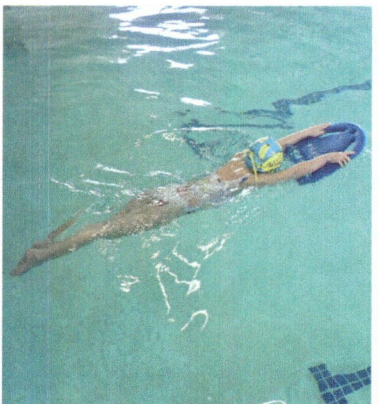

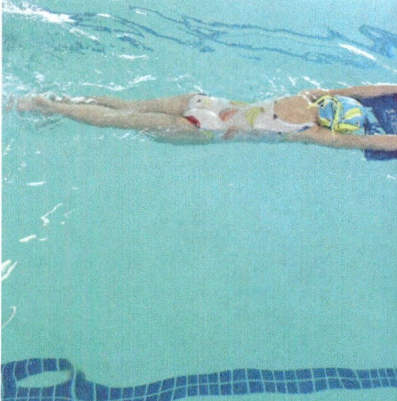

Skill 5: Kicks on the Side

Students start in a glide position, Flutter Kicking with their hips, leading with their left arm, rotating their body with their hips and right arm pulling down to the right side.

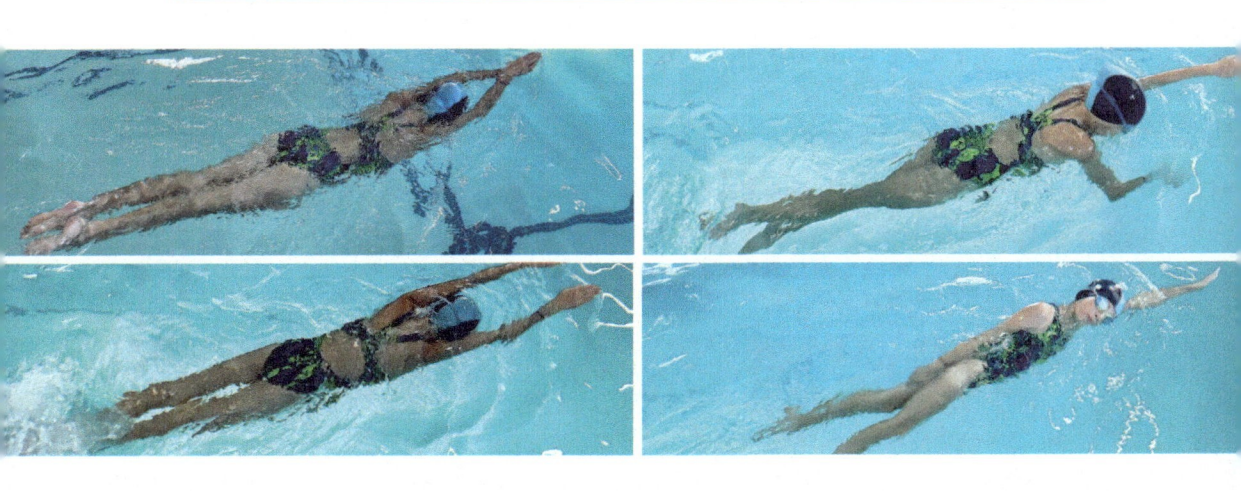

Skill 6: One Arm (Elbow, Breath, Reach)

Students learn how to rotate their bodies, pulling with their forearm, bringing their elbow up to the ceiling, sneaking in a perfect breath, and lastly reaching their arm out against their ear with fingers pointing to the bottom of the pool. LSI's method for timing is *elbow, breath, reach*.

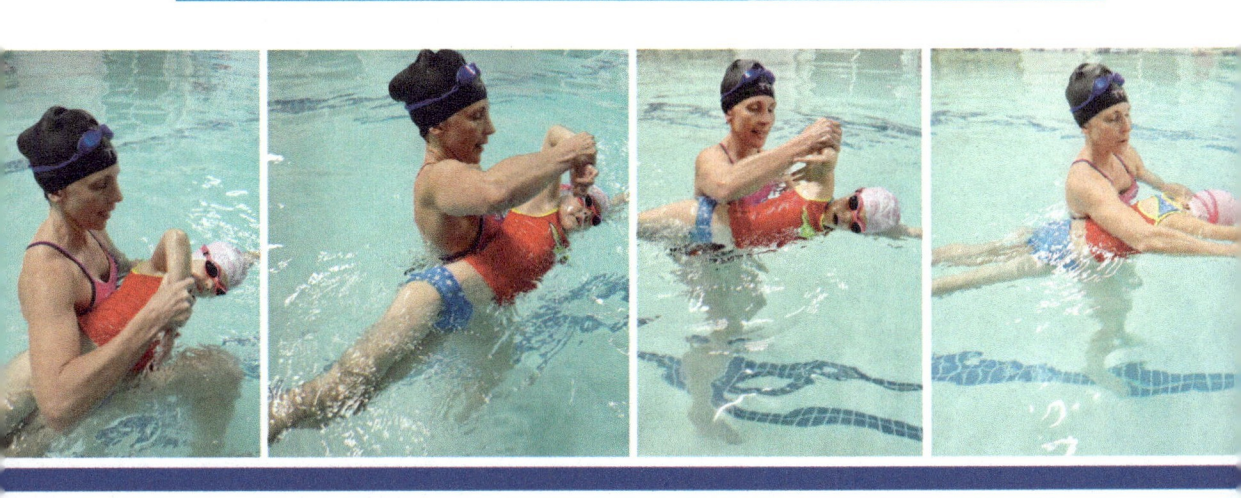

LSI SKILLS #2

Skill 7: Freestyle

Students learn their second stroke, which is their first competitive stroke, by continuing to build on the One Arm stroke. They add in the left arm, mirroring what they learned with the right arm, keeping their head down while still rotating and kicking from their hips.

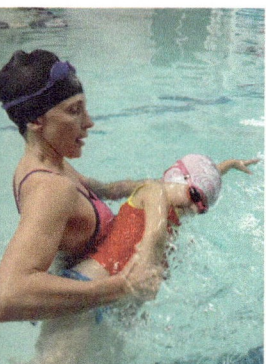

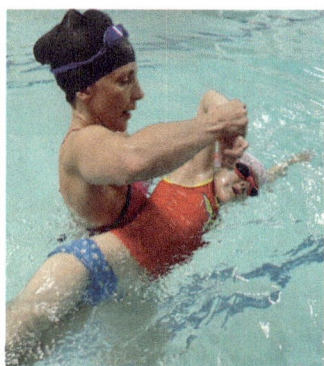

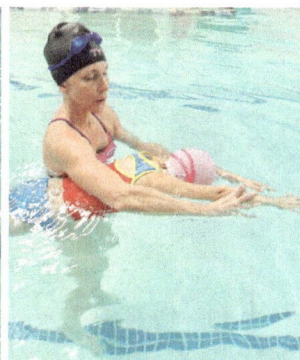

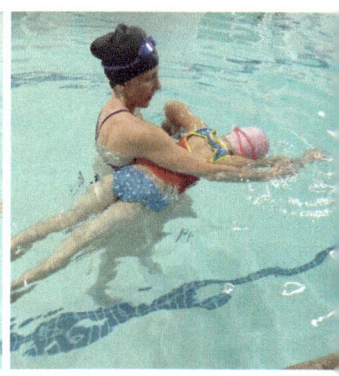

Skill 8: Kneeling Dives

Students review their sitting dives and move on to kneeling dives. This teaches them to push up with their back foot and out with the front foot, which helps them push their body forward and not down. Their arms remain behind their ears during the whole dive, keeping their chin down and their eyes looking back at the wall as they enter the water. Toes come together and point, making the perfect dive.

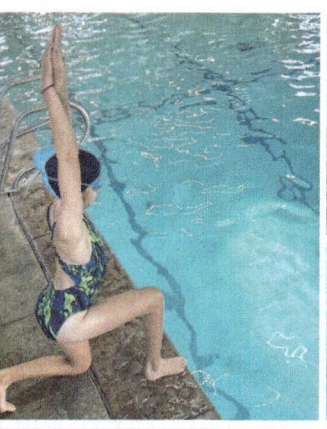

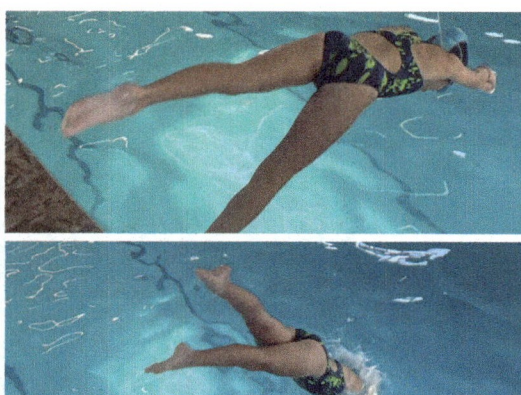

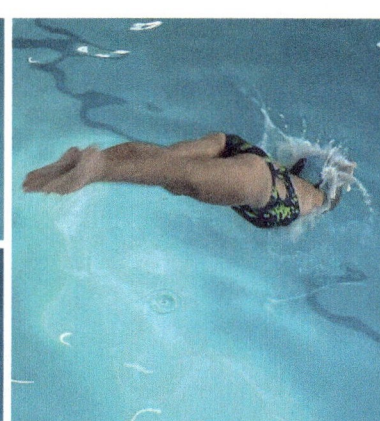

LIFESTYLE SWIMMING INSTRUCTION

Skill 9: Standing Dives

Students will move into standing dives after they have gotten comfortable with sitting and kneeling dives. They will learn to curl toes at the edge of pool, with only knees bent, making a "rainbow" or arch above and over the water, keeping their chin down and eyes looking back at the wall as they enter the water. Their toes should be together and pointed after they push off.

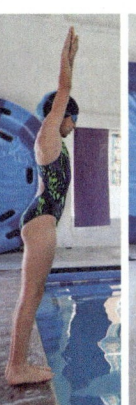

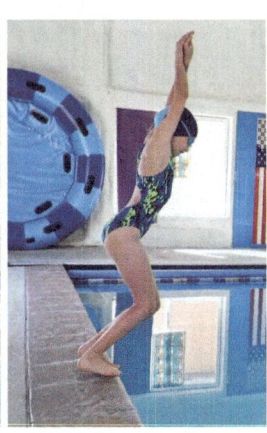

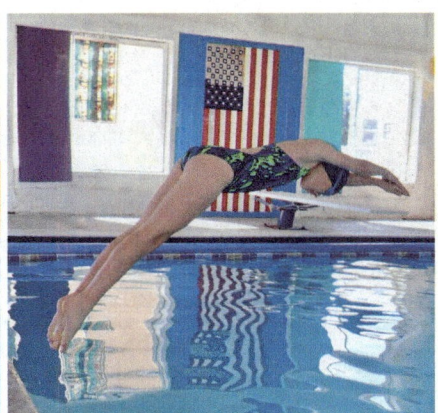

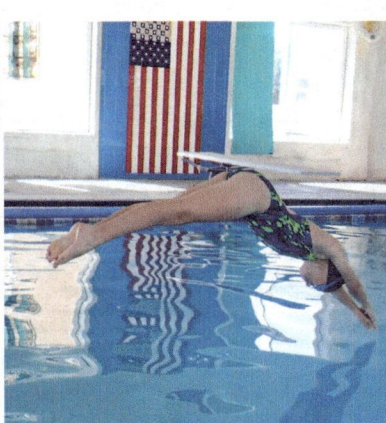

LSI SKILLS #2 PARTING SHOTS

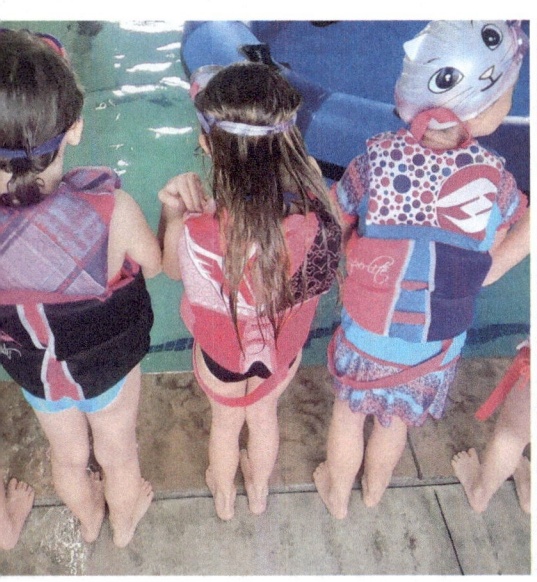

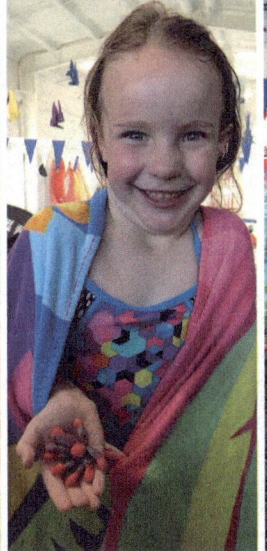

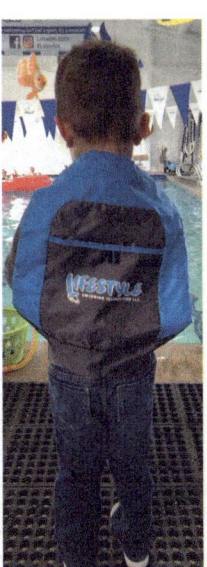

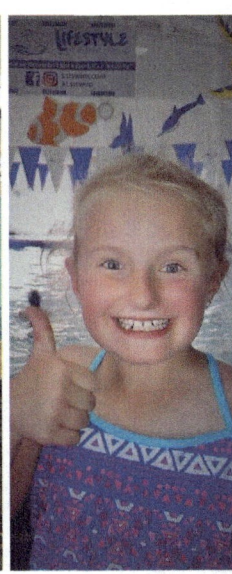

5

LSI SKILLS #3

Lanette came to LSI frustrated with her kids' previous swim lessons. She had been sending them to swim lessons for many years but saw that they still didn't have the confidence or ability to swim. After only six lessons with LSI, her children actually learned to swim. In other lessons they were still panicking in the water and she didn't feel comfortable with their abilities. They are now much safer in the water. Lanette was impressed with how the instructors taught the kids water safety and confidence. She loved the learning environment at LSI.

LSI Skills #3 is the third group class, and this class instills the importance of drills and technique before speed. Students who are familiar with all drills up to this point will look smoother in the water compared to students who have not been taught the correct body positions. In this class, students begin to learn how to do laps in the water and let the water work with their bodies instead of against them. Students work on a lot of drills in and out of the water. They will learn all dives in this class, start to work on flip turns, perfect their Freestyle, and begin the drills for Backstroke and Breaststroke.

Pre-Skills

Students must either graduate from LSI Skills #2 or know how to comfortably tread in any depth of water with head above the water and swim Freestyle with little help.

Skills #3

Skill 1: Kicks on Front and Back

Students will work on kicking from their hips on their front and back in a Streamline position, while getting comfortable in both positions with and without a kickboard.

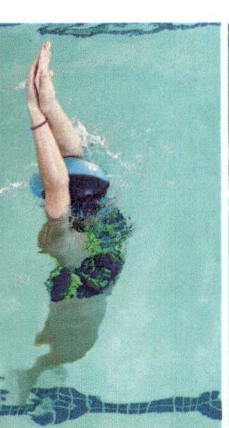

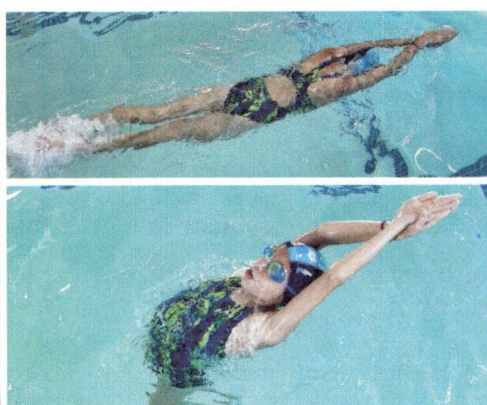

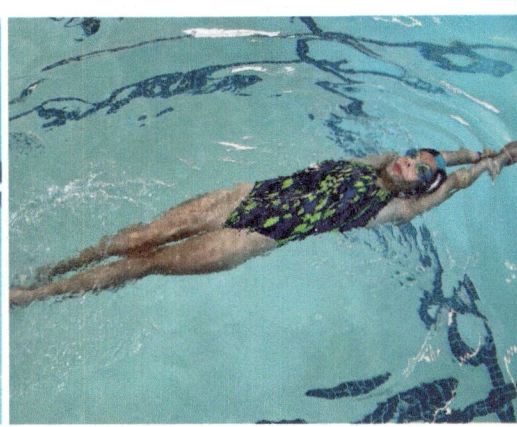

Skill 2: Perfecting Freestyle Drills

Practice makes perfect! Students will continue working on perfecting their Freestyle, maintaining technique with speed. They will start lap swimming more and will be corrected as needed. Repetition is required to get the student's stroke looking and feeling great.

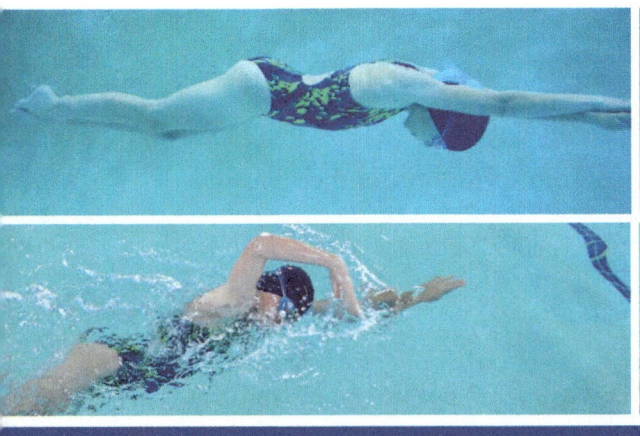

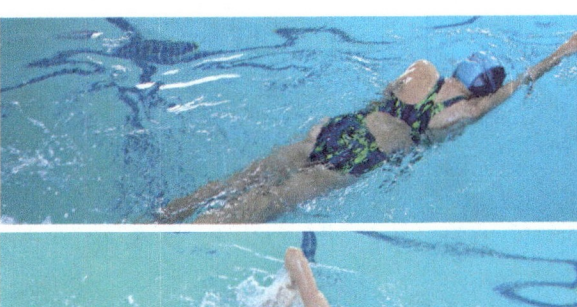

LSI SKILLS #3

Skill 3: Beginning Shoulder-to-Chin for Backstroke

This is a drill to understand the rotation of hips for both Freestyle and Backstroke. The student's whole body will rotate side to side with their hips while their head remains stationary, eyes looking up to the ceiling, and rotating enough for each shoulder to meet the chin on each side while Flutter Kicking.

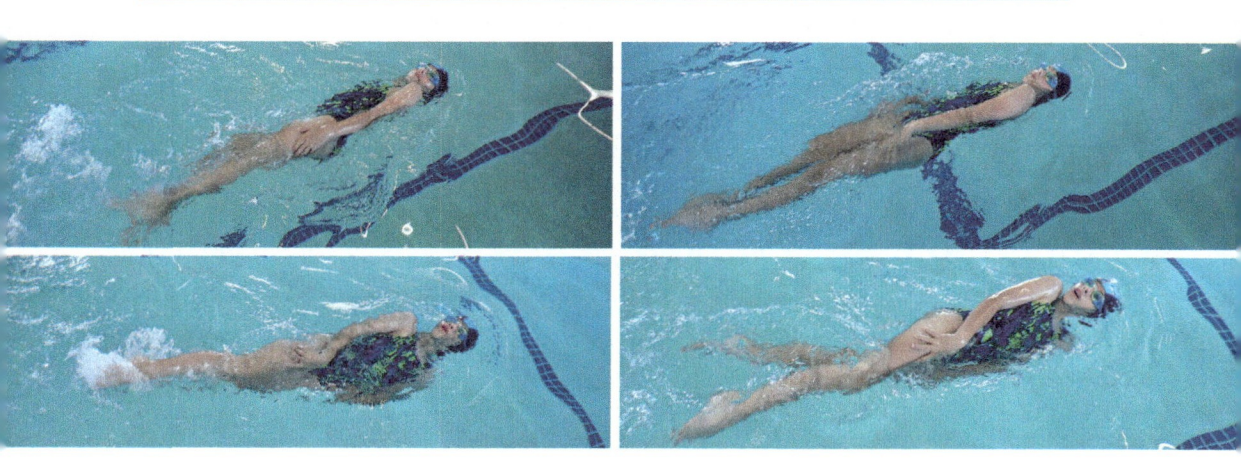

Skill 4: Learning Backstroke

Backstroke is the second competitive stroke. This stroke is taught right after Freestyle to teach the similarities between the two, making Backstroke easier to learn. Students will learn to keep their hips up, head stationary, arms reaching, and Flutter Kicking with hips while swimming this stroke.

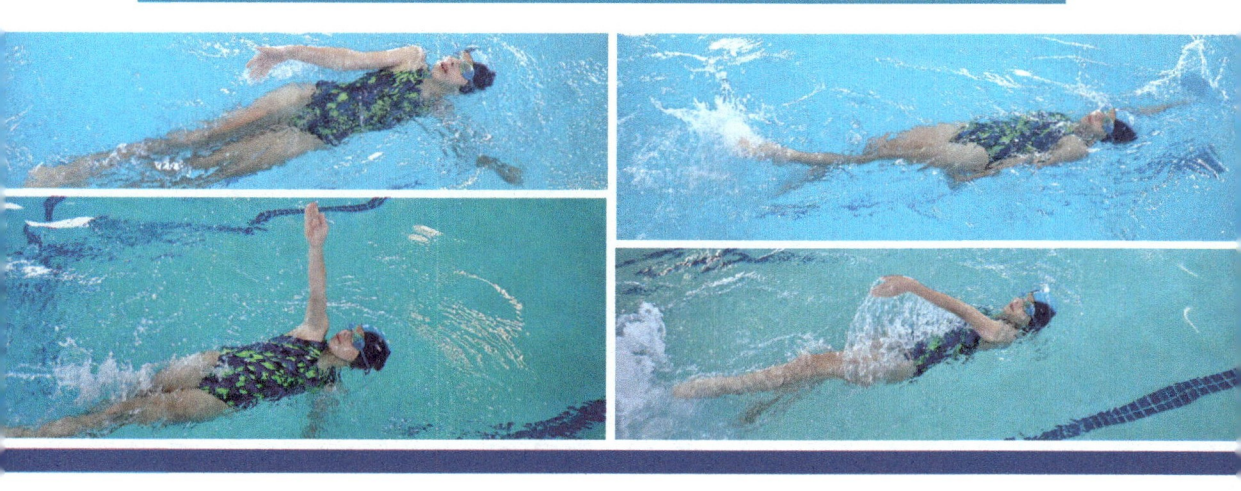

LIFESTYLE SWIMMING INSTRUCTION

Skill 5: Flip Turns

Students will learn to approach the wall by looking at the line at the bottom of the pool and timing their body to flip at the perfect time to push off the wall and continue swimming Freestyle.

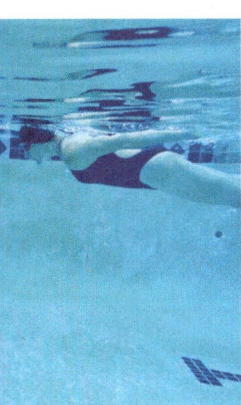

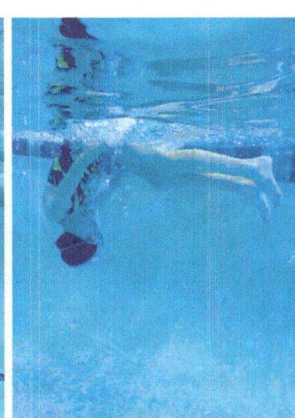

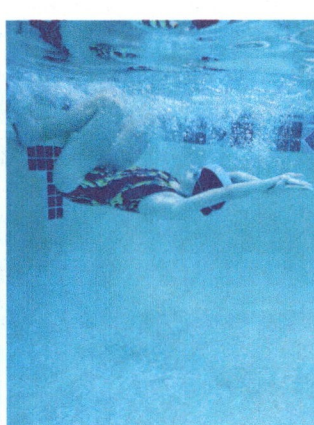

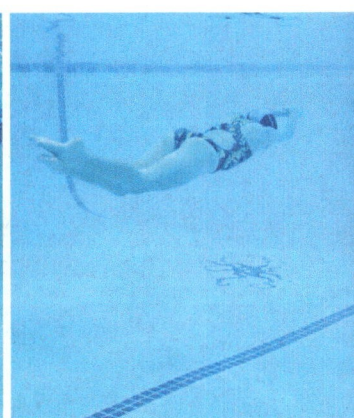

Skill 6: Starting Dives

Students will learn how to start their stroke off a starting block for Freestyle and learn how to do a Backstroke starting dive from the stainless-steel bar on the starting block.

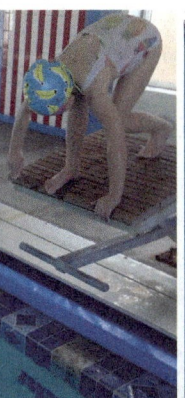

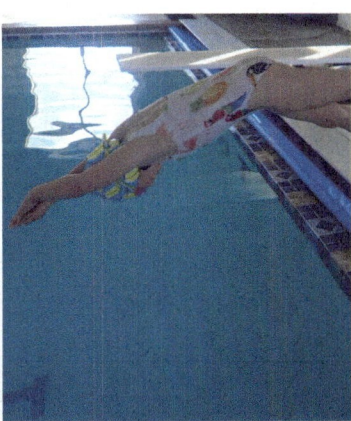

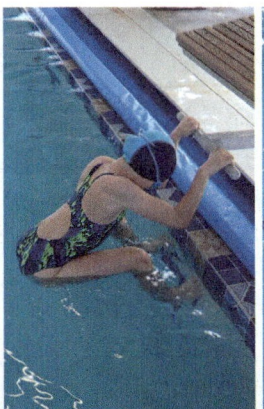

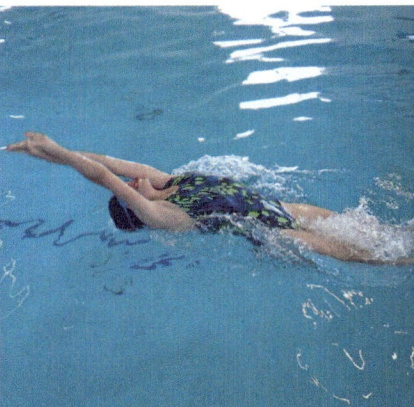

44

LSI SKILLS #3

LSI SKILLS #3 PARTING SHOTS

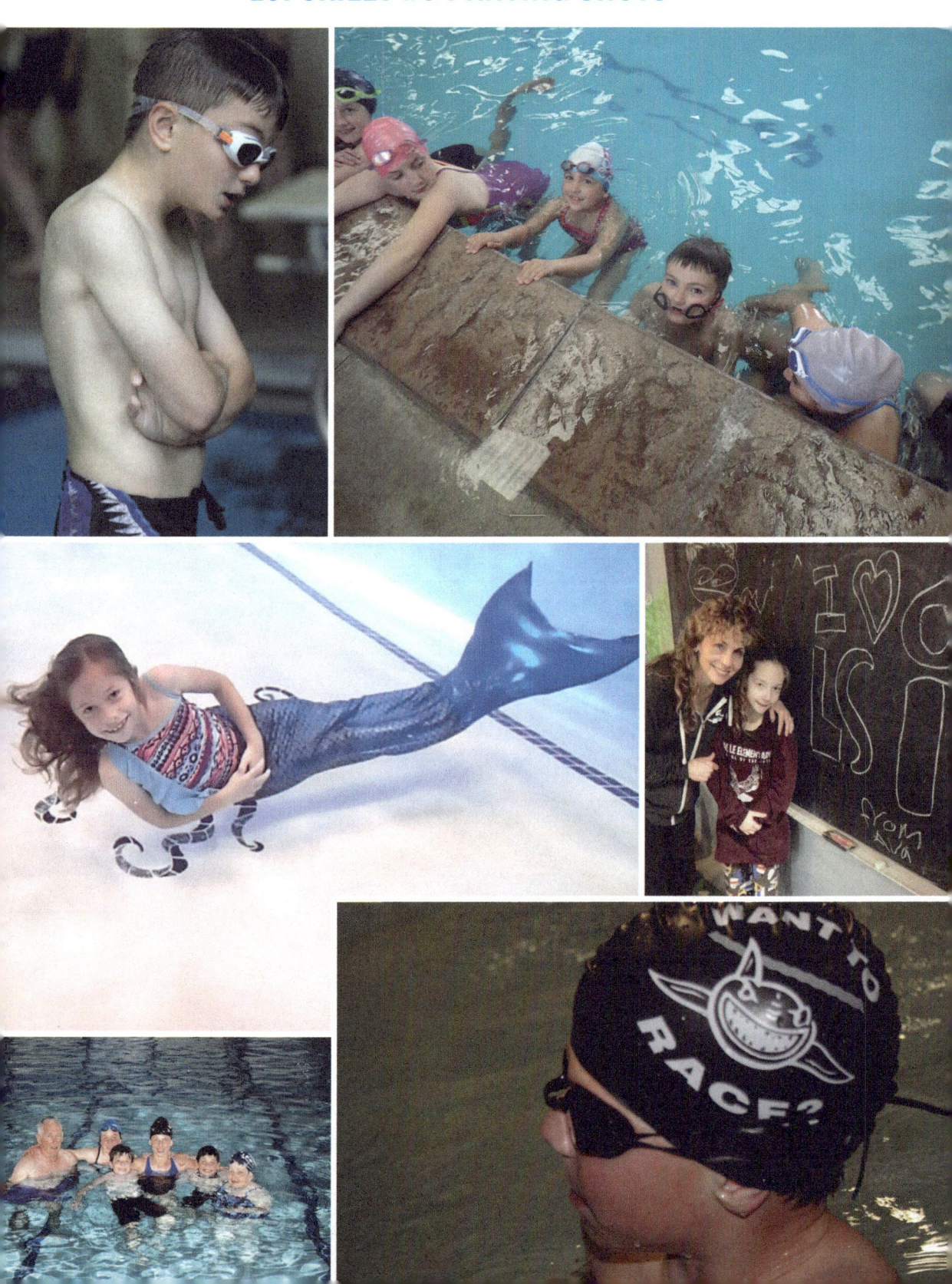

NOTES

6

LSI SKILLS #4

Savannah had been taking lessons at LSI for a number of years. One summer, she wanted to go to swim lessons with her cousins elsewhere. Her mom signed her up for the lessons. After the first lesson, Savannah's mom received a phone call from the instructor who ran the program. She needed to talk about Savannah. She told Savannah's mom that she felt guilty taking her money for lessons. She explained that Savannah was better than the three instructors she had in the pool teaching that first day. She asked what swim team Savannah was on and was told that she's not on a team but has been training to be on one. She asked about where Savannah normally takes lessons because her technique in all the swimming styles was better than anyone she had seen, especially for a 10-year-old. Savannah's mom told her about LSI. The woman was so impressed she gave Savannah a week at no charge because she didn't have an instructor on staff who would be able to improve Savannah's skill. LSI had taught her such good form, technique, and safety that by 10 years old, she had surpassed some instructors' abilities.

LSI Skills #4 is the fourth group class that continues to instill the importance of drills and technique before speed. In this class, students start treading with hands up and out of the water and review all previous competitive strokes. In this level the students will practice more, like they would if they were on a team. Lap swimming, warm-ups, and flip turns are expected. However, we still help students with technique if we see it is not perfect.

LIFESTYLE SWIMMING INSTRUCTION

In this class students will work on drills for Breaststroke and Butterfly, perfect their Streamline after their flip turns, and learn open turns for Breaststroke and Butterfly.

Pre-Skills

Students must either graduate from LSI Skills #3 or be fluid in Freestyle and Backstroke.

Skills #4

> **Skill 1: Treading With Hands Up**
>
> Students learn how to tread with no hands. This helps them to relax their legs and learn not to work so hard in the water.

> "SWIMMING IS NORMAL FOR ME. I'M RELAXED. I'M COMFORTABLE, AND I KNOW MY SURROUNDINGS. IT'S MY HOME.
>
> — MICHAEL PHELPS

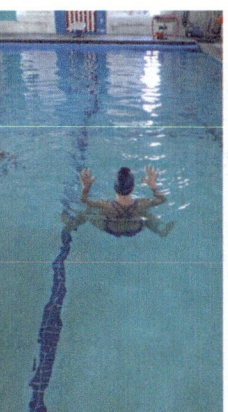

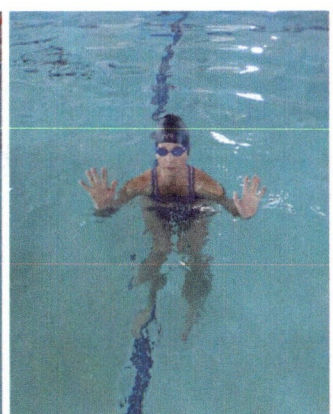

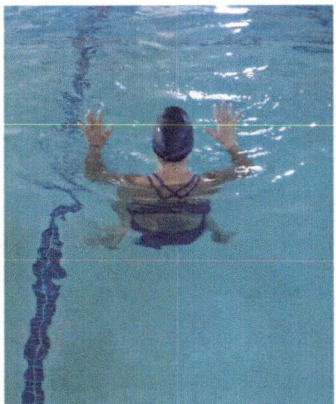

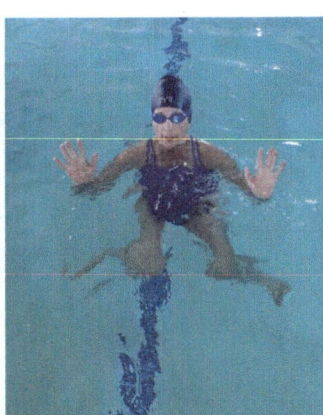

LSI SKILLS #4

Skill 2: Streamline for Freestyle and Backstroke

Students will learn to stretch their arms out as in a dive position, with arms behind their ears, and Dolphin Kick from their hips with toes touching. They will be on their front for Freestyle and Butterfly. They will learn that the more flexible they are in their feet, the less their knees will bend. Students will learn to Dolphin Kick on their back for Backstroke.

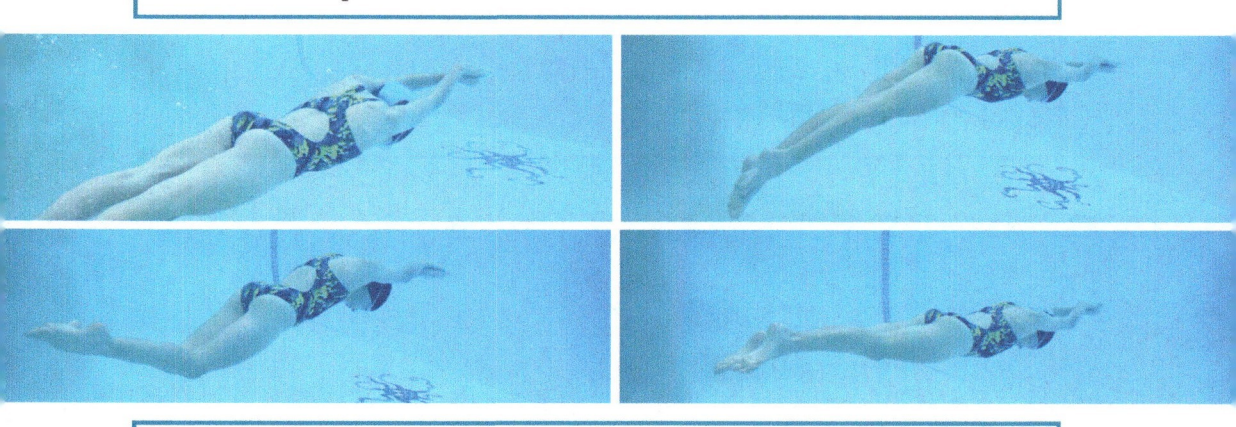

Skill 3: Breaststroke

This is the third competitive stroke. Students will start in a glide position and end in a glide position with hands and feet together. The arms pull under the water, forearms pulling the water back with elbows up high. Students make a scoop, shaped like an upside-down heart, and slice it down the middle. This will help bring the head forward and up to take a quick breath as the legs do a Whip Kick and Glide (pull, breath, kick, glide).

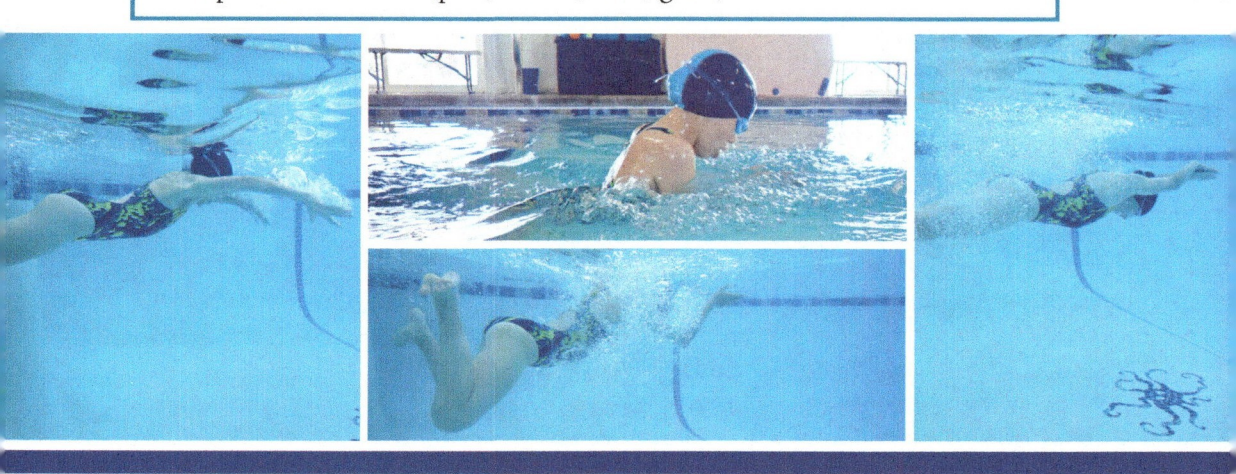

Skill 4: Underwater Pullout

In Breaststroke, a pullout is used instead of a Streamline. From a dive or push off the wall, hands and feet stay together. Using the momentum from the dive or push, students do a Dolphin Kick first and then a pull down with arms, hands placed on thighs. Rounding the back will help bring students to the surface. Students will then do a quick sneak pull with a Whip Kick following under the water before doing the first actual Breaststroke on top of the water (pull, breath, kick, glide).

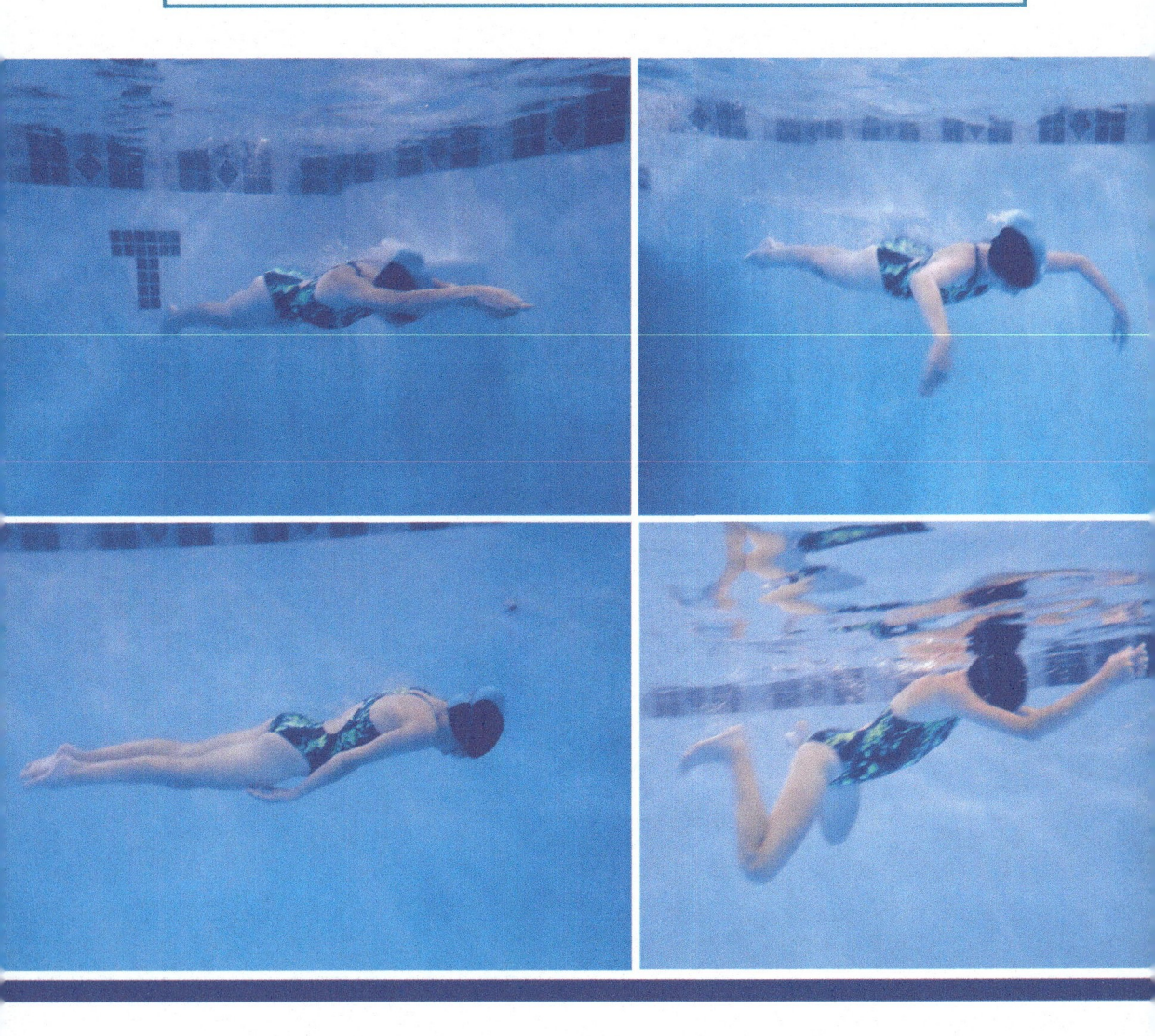

Skill 5: Butterfly (Fly)

This is the fourth and last competitive stroke. From a Streamline position, the student will Dolphin Kick and pull both arms under the water at the same time. When arms come out of the water by their hips, they will Dolphin Kick again, taking a quick breath before they fly their arms like butterfly wings, getting their head down before their arms come back into the water extending from their shoulders, forming another pull with fingernails down. A breath does not need to be taken every time. Timing in this stroke is crucial. Dolphin Kick from the hips with toes touching the whole time, undulating legs in a wave-like motion, forming two kicks per stroke to the beat *kick, kick, fly*.

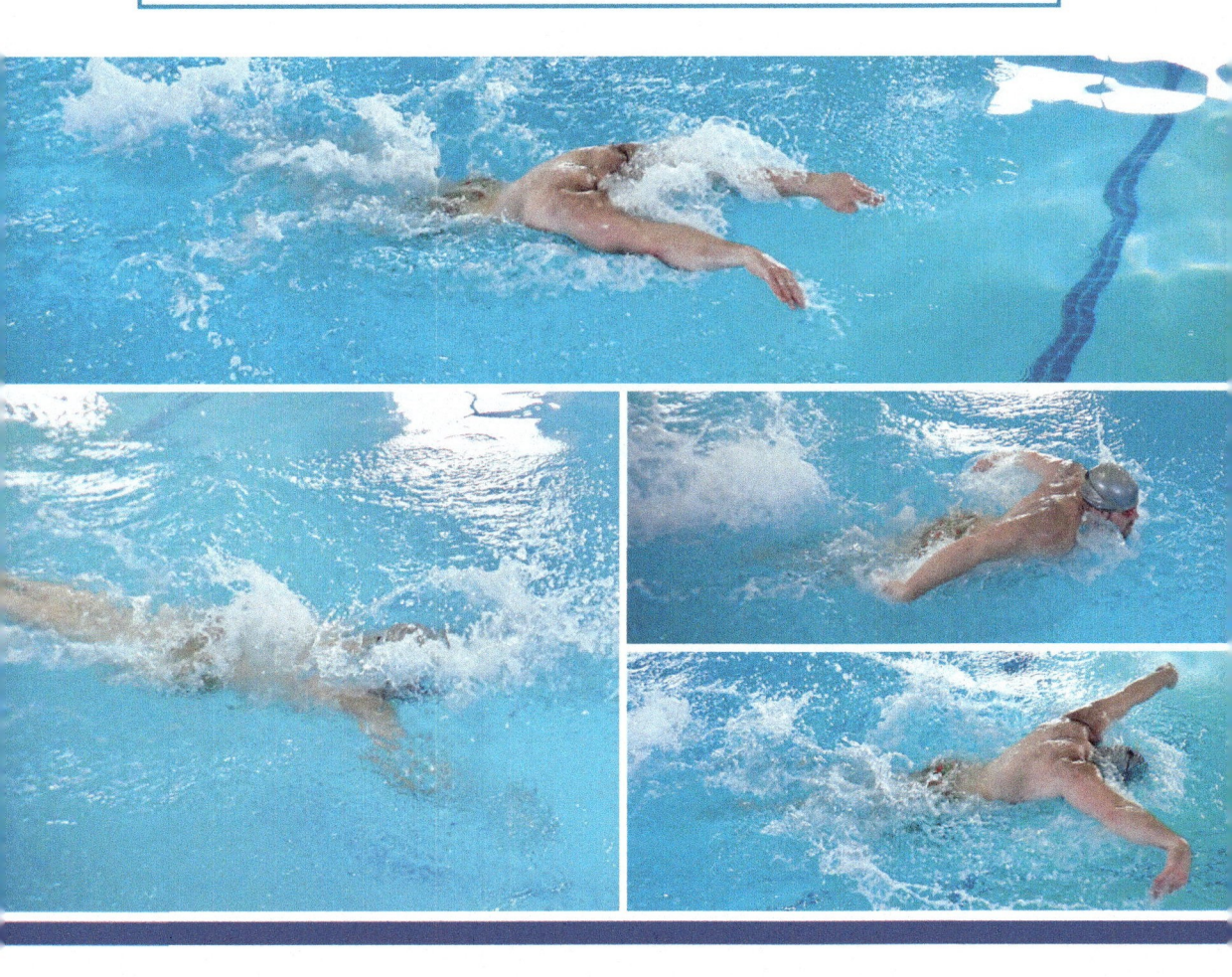

LIFESTYLE SWIMMING INSTRUCTION

> **Skill 6: Open Turns**
>
> Students learn to approach the wall with a two-hand touch for Breaststroke and Butterfly, sinking one elbow in the water, pushing with both feet on the wall, sinking hips down, and reaching the other arm over in the water, then doing an underwater pullout for Breaststroke or a Streamline for Butterfly.

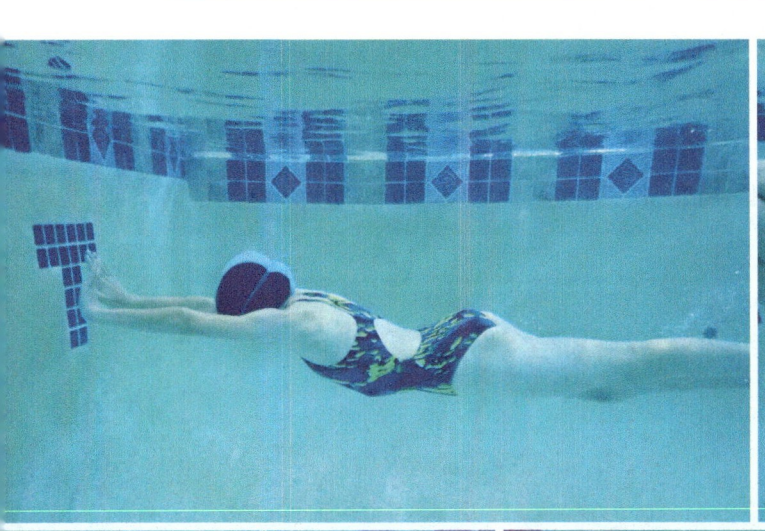

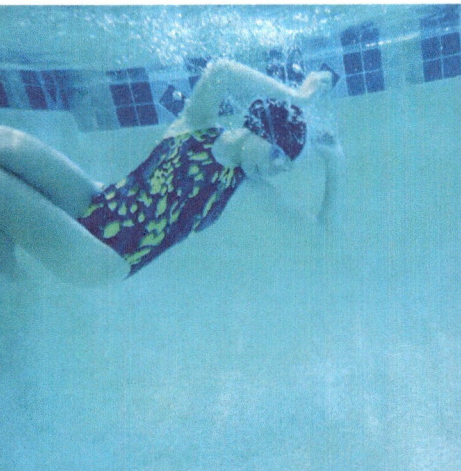

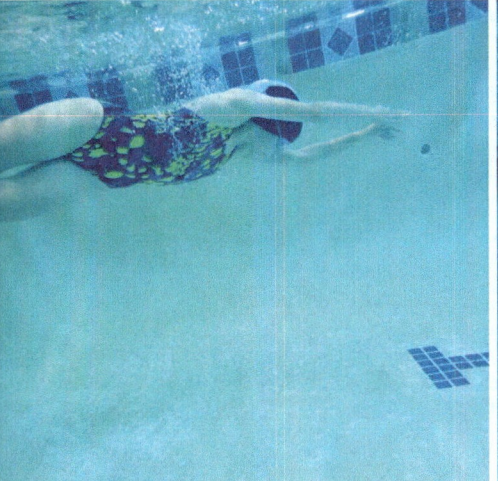

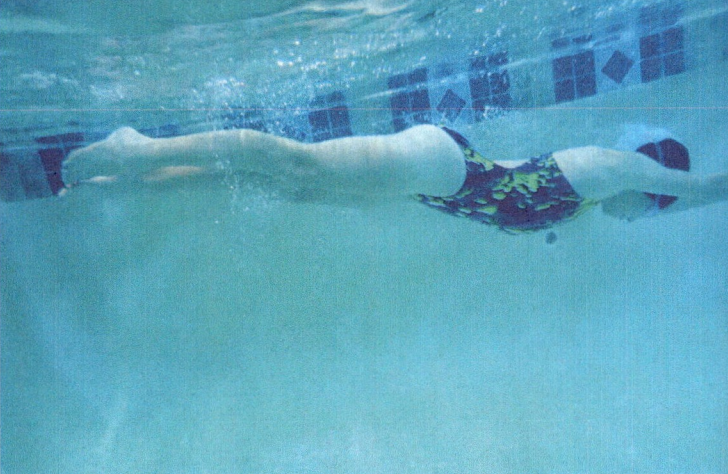

LSI SKILLS #4 PARTING SHOTS

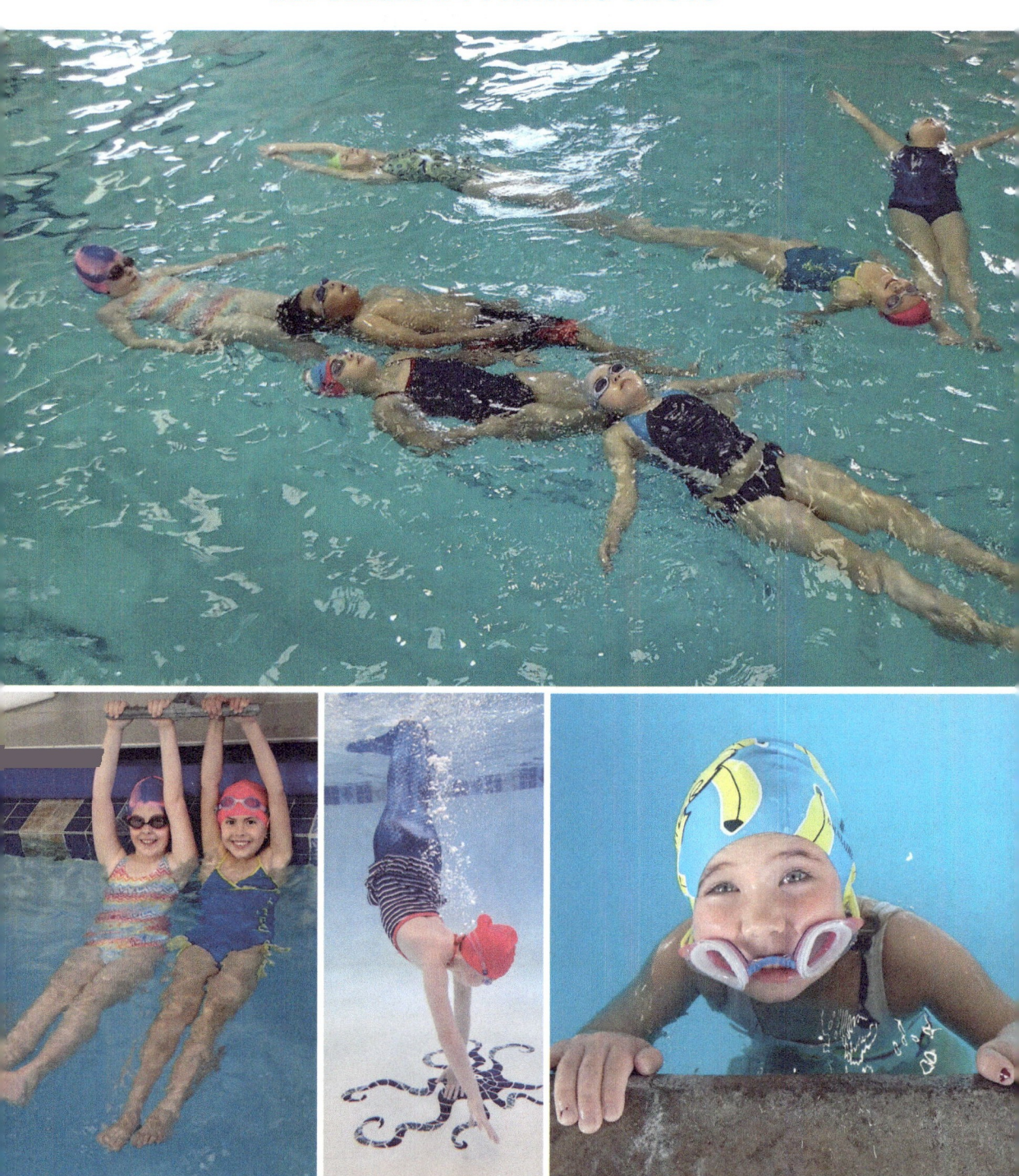

NOTES

7

LSI CLINICS: SWIM TEAM PREP

Jana and Jeff believed that knowing how to swim was a must for their children. They enrolled their children in Baby Beginnings at LSI. It didn't take long for them to come to love LSI's creative instruction and focus on technique. The skills the children learned in each class level built upon skills learned in the previous level. Their daughter struggled with a fear of going underwater and frequently cried. She fought any attempt to get her to float on her back or put her face in the water. The instructors were patient and encouraging with her. Through LSI's program, she gained confidence and grew to love swimming. She even aspired to join the swim team. At age 8½, she tried out for the YMCA swim team. The coach asked where she learned how to swim since she stood out amongst the others trying out that day. Her parents attribute her success to the foundation and focus on technique that she received in her five-plus years of lessons at LSI.

Swim Team Prep Clinic is a group class for students who need extra help to join a future swim team or extra coaching for their current swim team. Students practice all strokes, walls, starts, timing, and speed. They need to know their strokes before joining this class. This is a fast-paced class.

Pre-Skills

Students must either graduate from all LSI Skills classes, be training to join a swim team, or be on a swim team and need more technical coaching.

LIFESTYLE SWIMMING INSTRUCTION

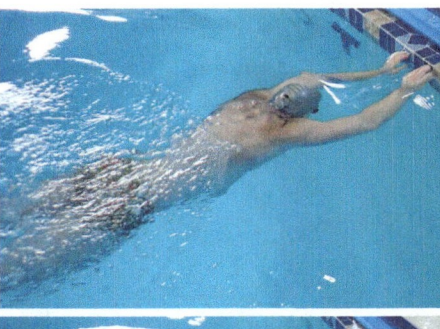

Swim Team Prep Skills

Skill 1: Starting Dives

Dives can't be practiced enough. The students practice a lot of dives, so they are the first ones off the block when they race and also dive the farthest.

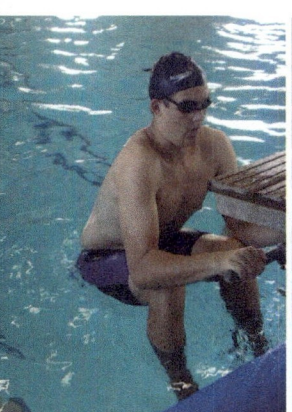

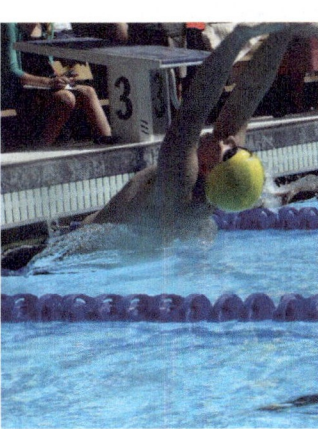

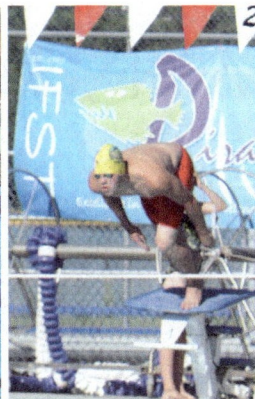

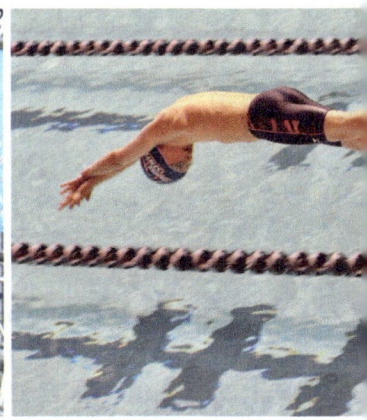

Skill 2: Faster Turns

Students work on timing walls better for flip turns and faster open turns.

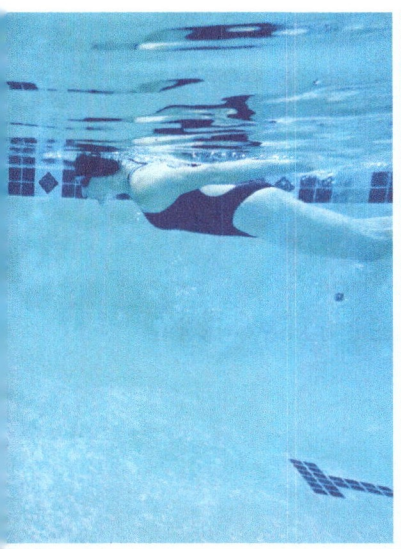

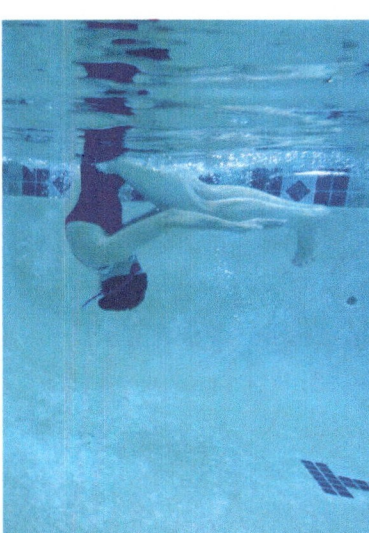

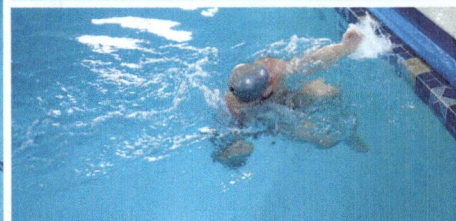

56

Skill 3: Streamline

Students work on longer and faster Streamline, arms staying behind their ears and head in line with their spine, and breathing on second stroke, not first.

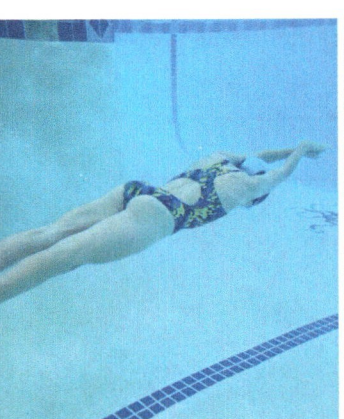

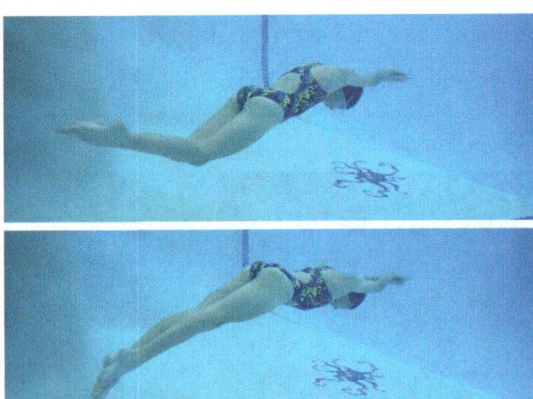

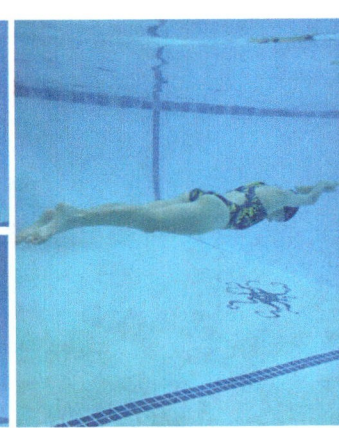

Skill 4: Working With Equipment to Improve Times

Students by now come ready to swim before class starts. Equipment is used for swimmers to learn how the water feels when everything is where it is supposed to be. Snorkels work on timing, paddles work on pull, and fins work on speed. Once their technique is where it is supposed to be, these tools add speed while keeping bodies fluid in the water.

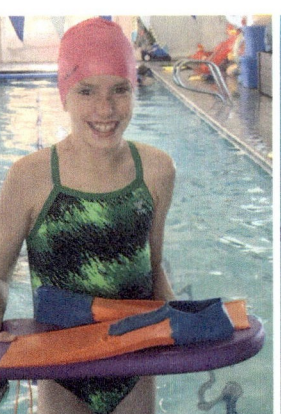

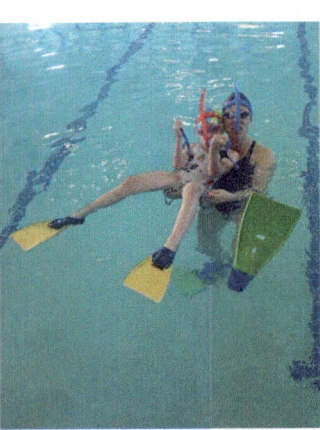

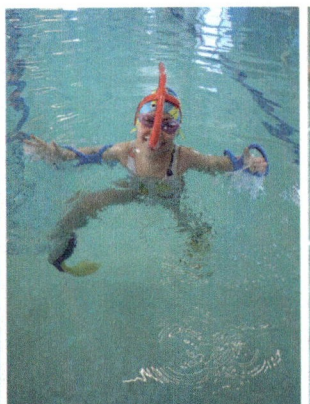

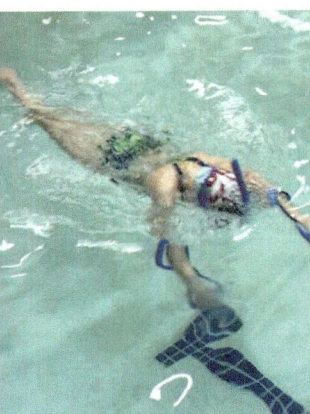

Skill 5: Race Time

Students learn to put all their training together. Technique before speed is how they train. This makes them race-ready so they do not have to think about technique while they race. LSI teaches them to get a better understanding of competition. They learn to hold their stroke together under pressure and when they are tired. And lastly, they learn to never give up!

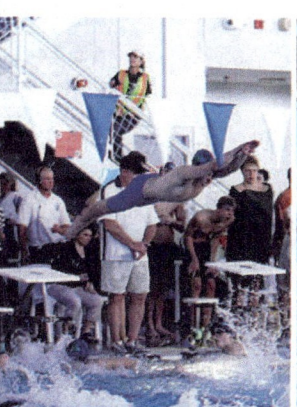

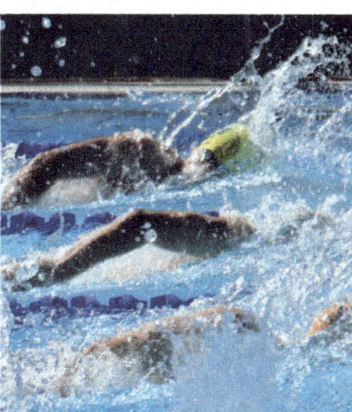

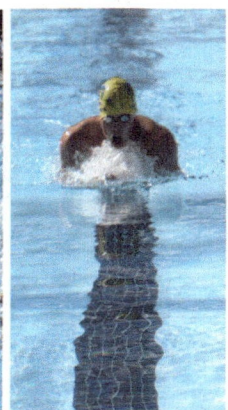

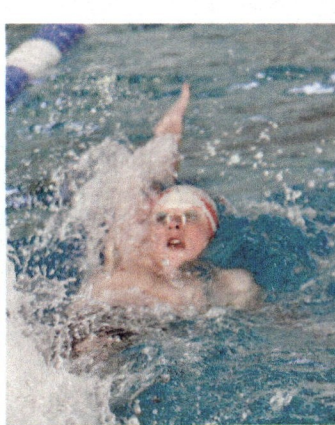

LSI CLINICS: SWIM TEAM PREP

STP PARTING SHOTS

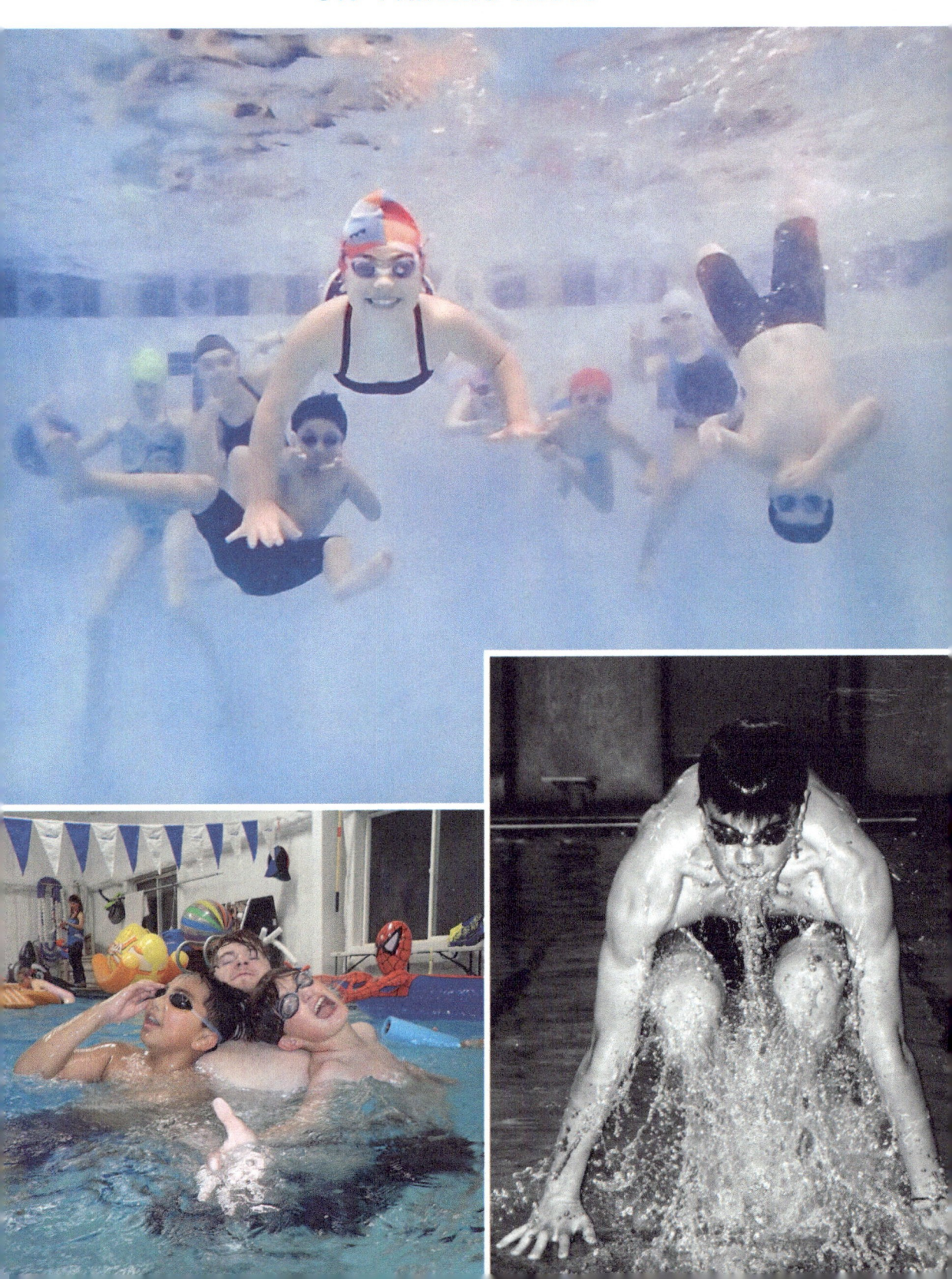

NOTES

8

LSI CLINICS: ADULT BEGINNERS

Yaneth always shied away when people discussed their adventures in water. She was in her 40s and had never learned to swim. Prior to joining Lifestyle Swimming Instruction, she had attempted to learn to swim as an adult from several instructors. None of those experiences provided the support she needed to successfully learn. Yaneth's first instructor never even got into the pool with her. After a few experiences of taking swim lessons and not learning how to swim, she had an increased fear of the water and a feeling of defeat. She first heard about LSI when she was in search of swim lessons for her 6-year-old son. When Yaneth found out that LSI offered multiple level adult classes, she did not hesitate to sign up. She quickly found that the instructors encouraged adults just like they did children. When Yaneth signed up for the class, she didn't believe that she would learn to swim. She thought that she might be able to float in water and get some exercise in the shallow portion of the pool, but she quickly found that LSI's goal was to teach her to swim and swim correctly. The LSI program built confidence in her ability to swim, the instructors were consistent and reliable, and the focus was to provide the students with the appropriate steps to move forward in their swim journey. She ended up inviting her older sister to join her in the adult swim class. Her sister learned to swim as well. They are both proud to say that they learned to swim in their 40s thanks to Lifestyle Swimming Instruction.

LIFESTYLE SWIMMING INSTRUCTION

Adult Clinic #1 is a group class for students 18-100-plus years old. Students graduate this class when they can float on front, back float, swim Elementary Backstroke, understand all Freestyle drills, swim Freestyle, and are comfortable in all depths of water.

Pre-Skills

Adults can join this class even if they have never put a foot in the water. They are separated by ability so each student can go at their own pace and get over their aquaphobia with strategic help.

LSI Beginning Adult Skills

Skill 1: Nose Bubbles

Students learn how to quickly go under the water by taking a breath above the water in through their mouth and out through their nose. This forms nose bubbles under the water, so no water goes up their nose and they do not inhale any water while going under.

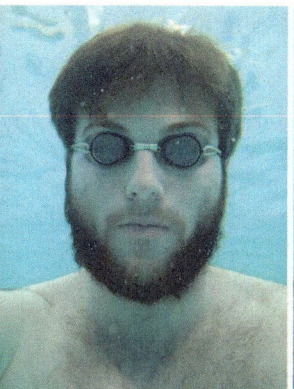

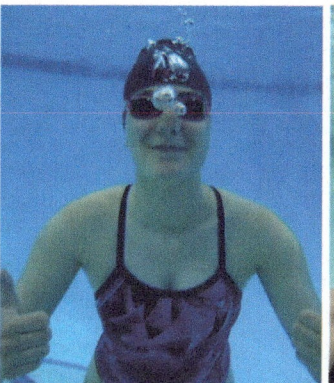

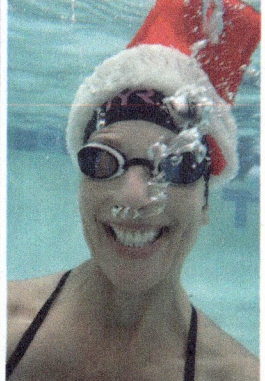

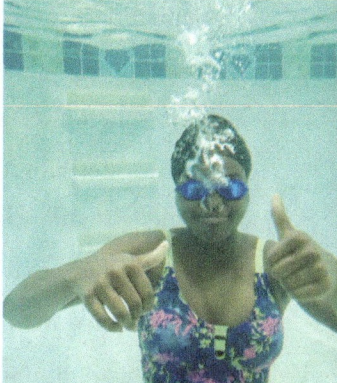

"IF YOU ALWAYS PUT LIMITS ON EVERYTHING YOU DO, PHYSICAL OR ANYTHING ELSE, IT WILL SPREAD INTO YOUR WORK AND INTO YOUR LIFE. THERE ARE NO LIMITS. THERE ARE ONLY PLATEAUS, AND YOU MUST NOT STAY THERE, YOU MUST GO BEYOND THEM."

— BRUCE LEE

LSI CLINICS: ADULT BEGINNERS

> ### Skill 2: Back Floats
> Students learn how to trust the water to hold them by floating on their back.

> ### Skill 3: Glides
> Students learn how the water helps move them when they are relaxed and their head is in line with their spine, with each arm touching each ear, parallel to each other, and toes touching.

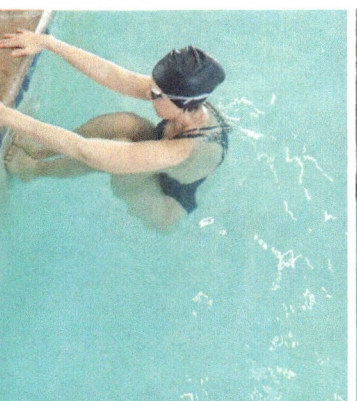

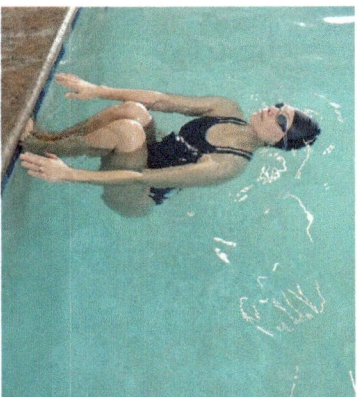

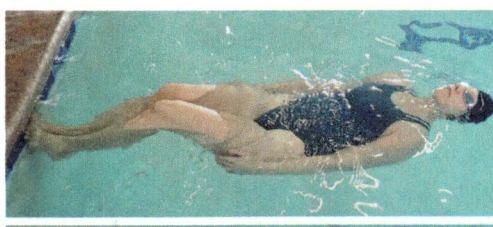

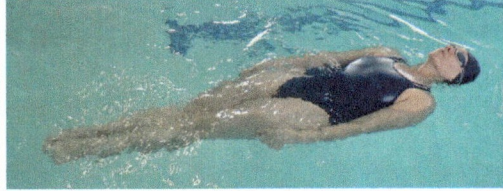

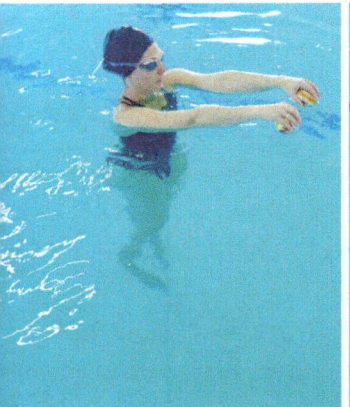

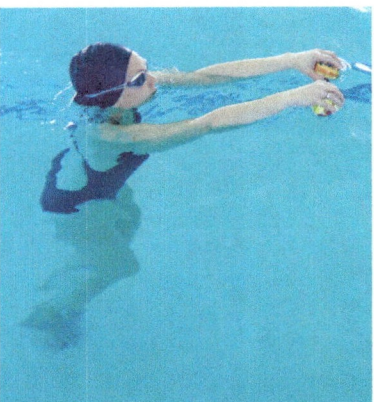

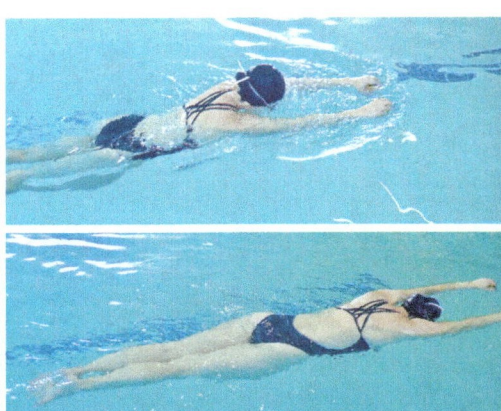

Skill 4: Glide-Reach-Roll

This is the foundational move for any skill. Students will glide for two seconds, keeping their left ear touching their left arm, pulling their right arm straight down to their side while rotating their hips and then ending up on their back.

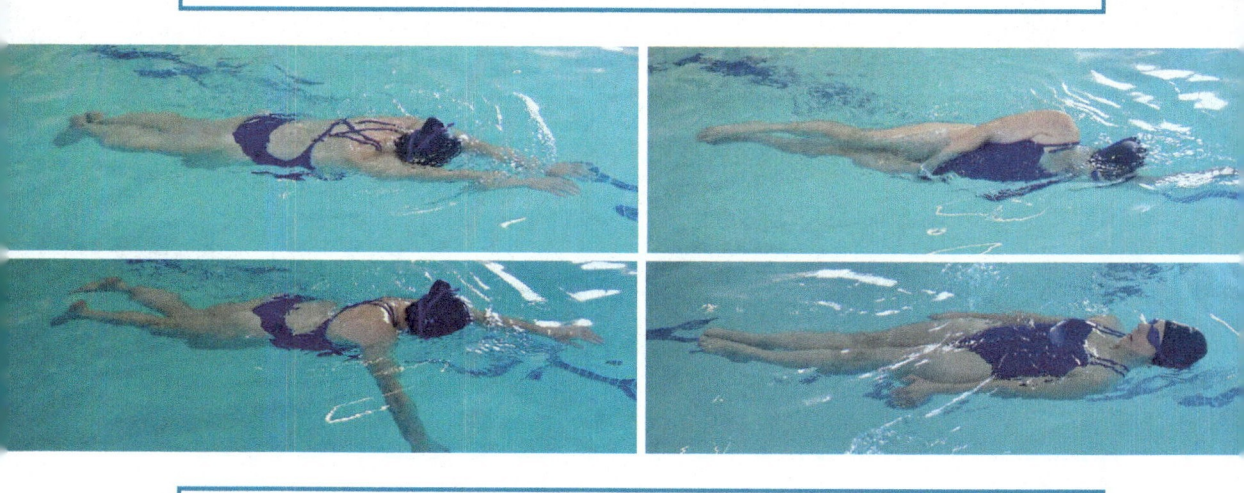

Skill 5: Elementary Backstroke

This is the first stroke adult students learn to get across the water. Starting with a back float, hands slide up each side while pushing with heels, drawing two half circles with toes, ending with toes touching to form a back glide. This creates the first kick, a Whip Kick.

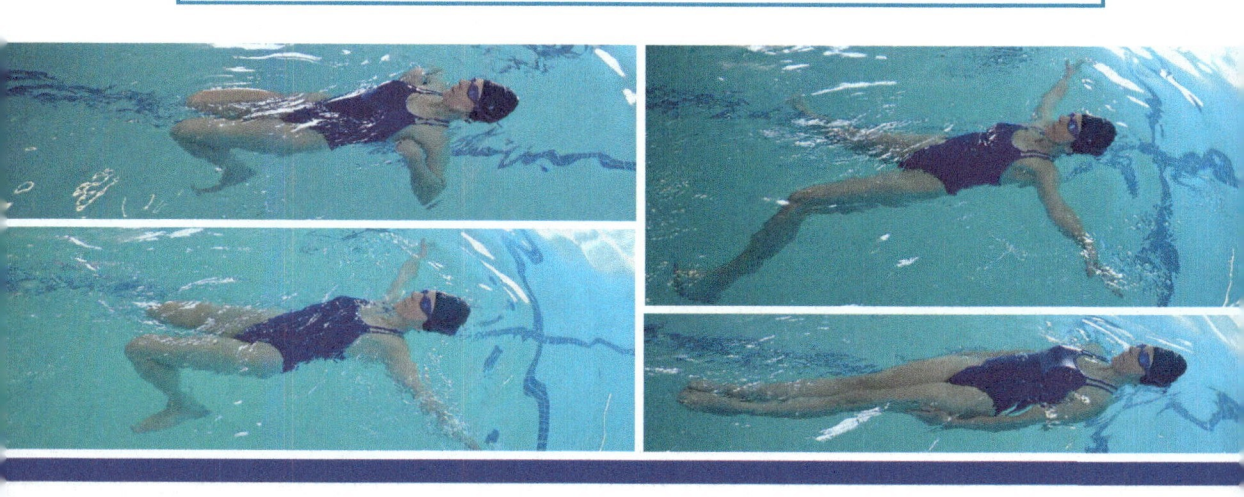

LSI CLINICS: ADULT BEGINNERS

Skill 6: Treads

Students learn to tread in the water by scooping their arms toward them while doing the Whip Kick that they have already been taught in Elementary Backstroke. They will learn to do this with their heads up in 10 feet of water, without help, once they graduate from this class.

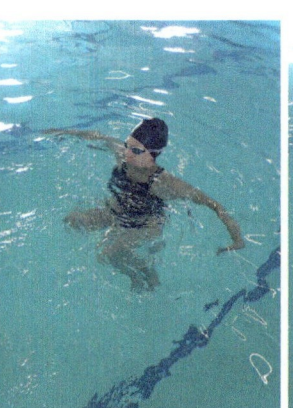

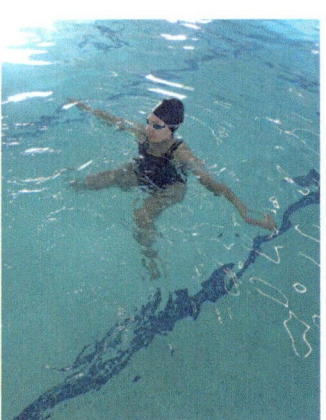

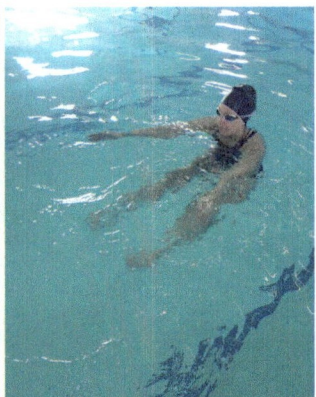

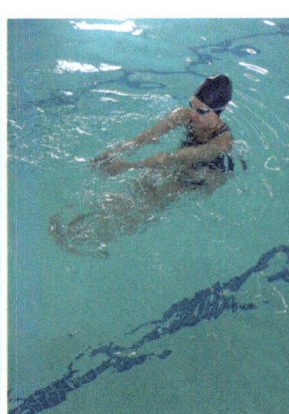

Skill 7: Deep Bobs

Adults learn to do bobs in at least 10 feet of water. This is a game changer with adults, especially for getting comfortable in deep water. It builds their confidence in being in any depth of water.

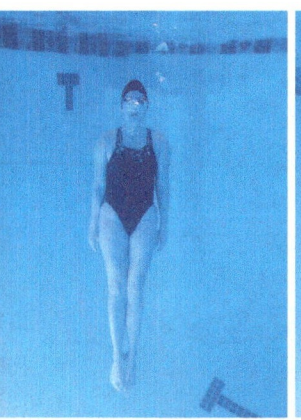

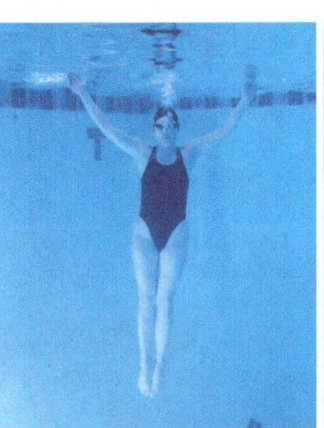

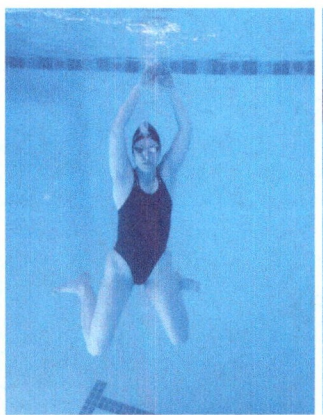

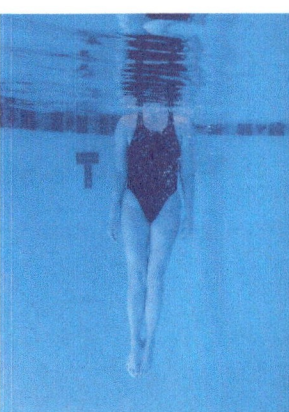

Skill 8: Flutter Kicks

Students do more kicking from their hips on their front and also on their back, now in a Streamline position, working on getting comfortable in both positions with and without a kickboard.

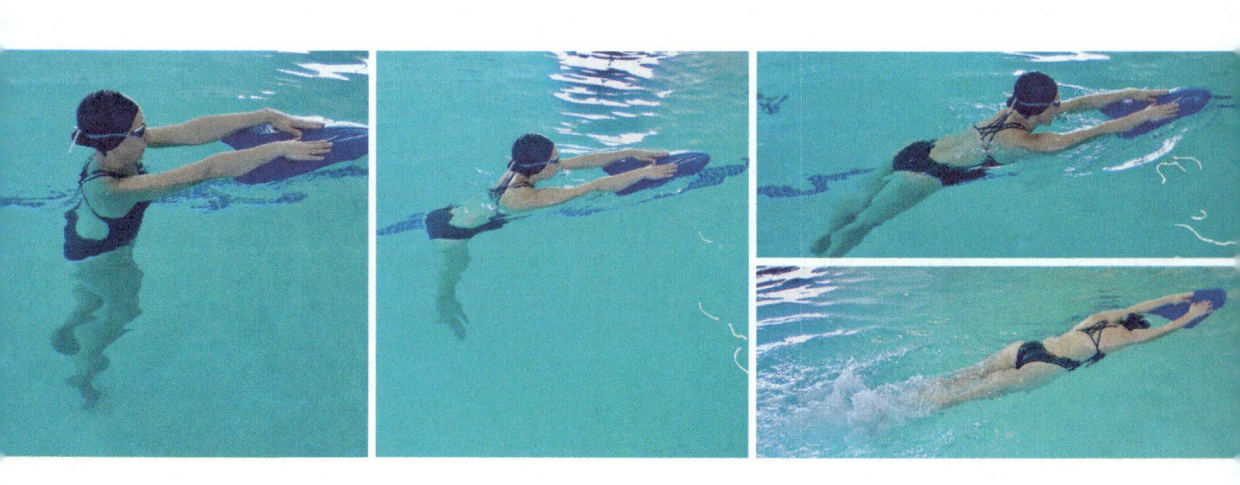

Skill 9: Kicking on Side

Students learn how to continue their kick from their hips, while learning to rotate their hips at the same time.

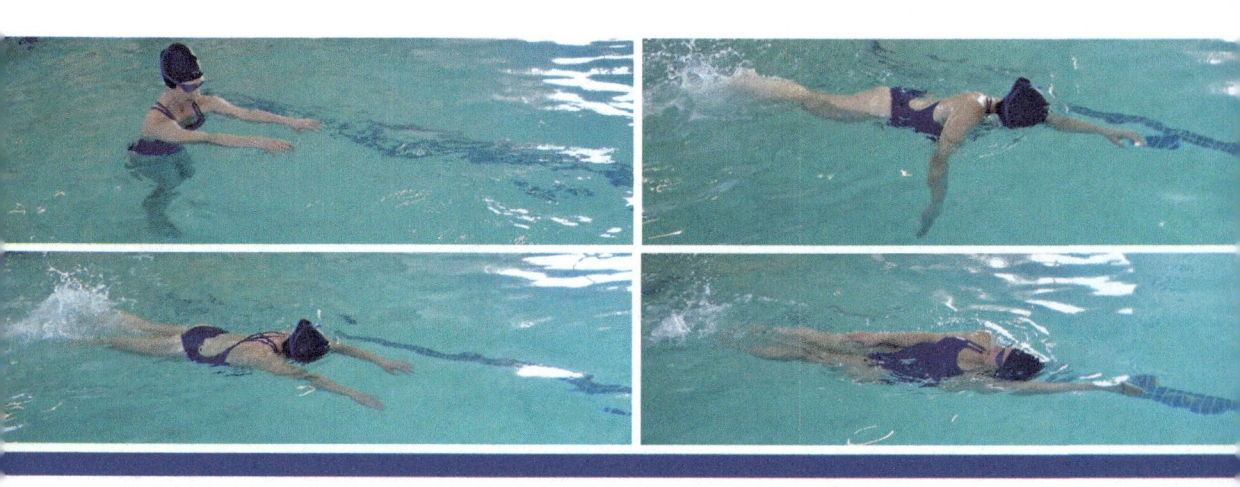

Skill 10: One Arm (Elbow, Breath, Reach)

Students learn how to rotate their bodies and pull with their forearm, bring their elbow up to the ceiling, sneak in a perfect breath, and reach that arm out on the ear with fingers pointing to the bottom of the pool (elbow, breath, reach).

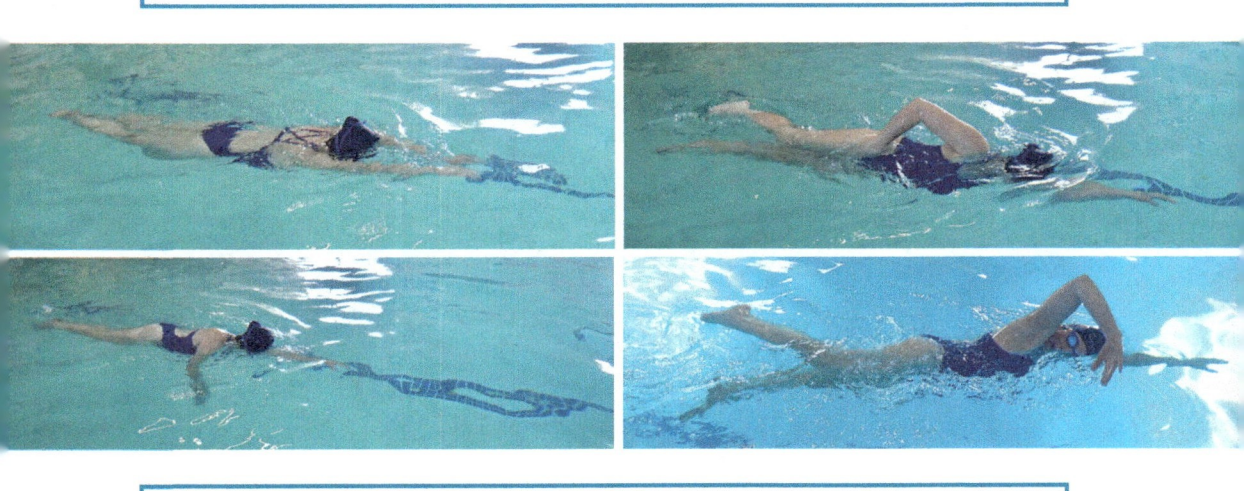

Skill 11: Freestyle

Students learn their second stroke. This stroke is their first competitive stroke. They will continue the One Arm stroke, learning to make the same movement with their second arm, except they will learn to keep their head down on the second arm stroke while rotating their hips first and continuing kicks from their hips.

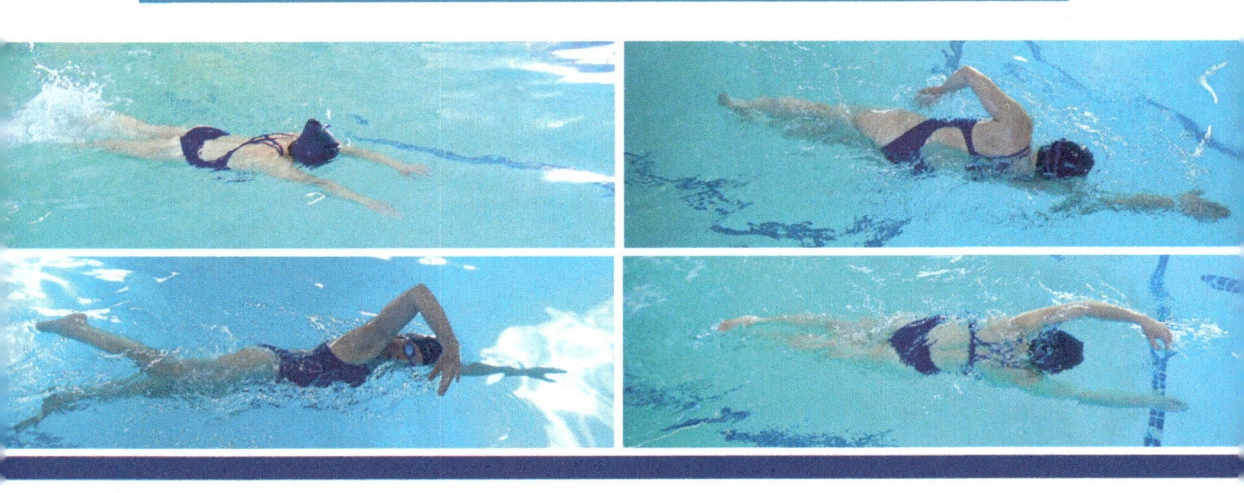

LIFESTYLE SWIMMING INSTRUCTION

> ### Skill 12: Jumping in Deep Water
> LSI's method to teach adults to jump into deep water is to curl their toes at edge of the pool and jump straight out in 10 feet of water, with assistance and spotting in the beginning.

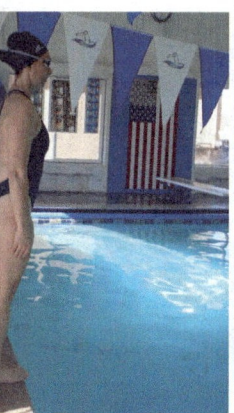

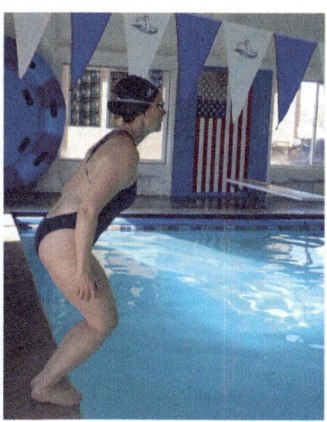

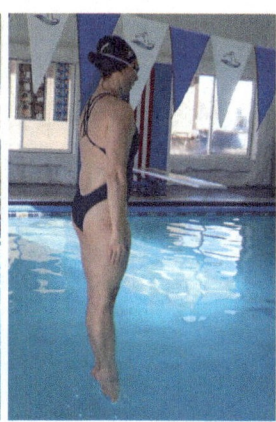

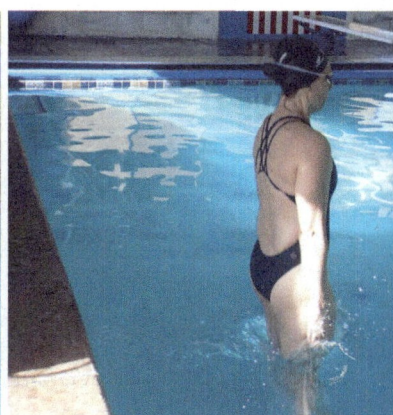

ADULT PARTING SHOTS

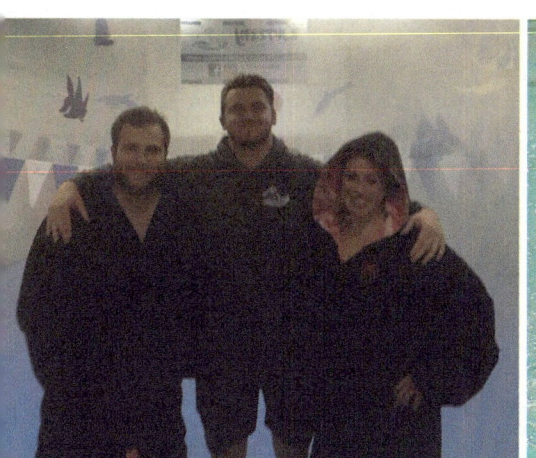

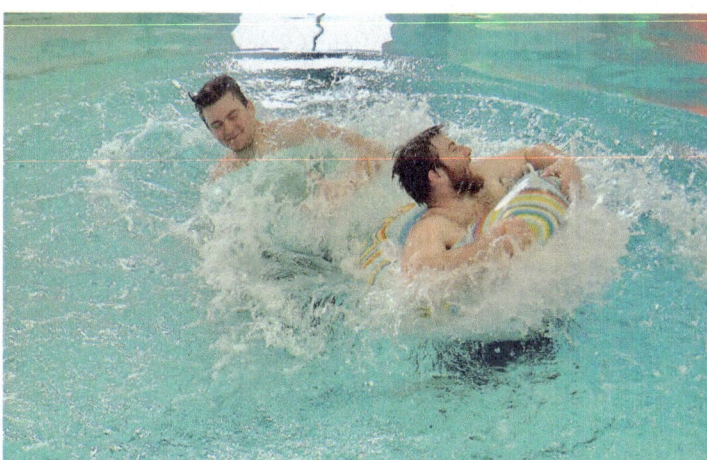

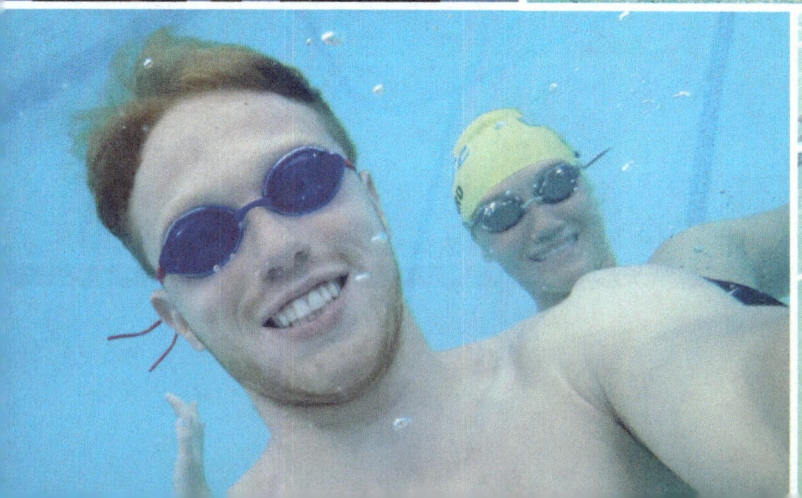

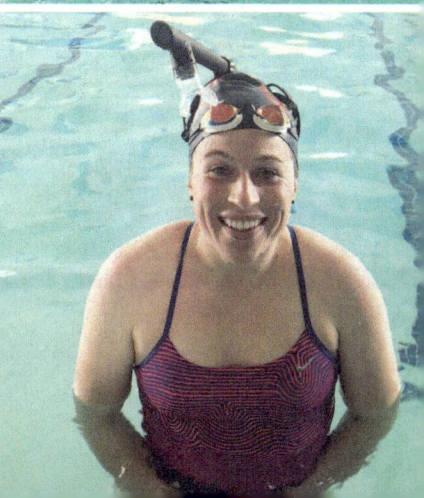

9

LSI CLINICS:
ADULT INTERMEDIATE AND ADVANCED

Amy tore her ACL while playing with her kids at a trampoline park. The injury ended up being a catalyst in correcting broken muscle chains in her body's movement. Between ACL rehabilitation (which required a year of physical therapy) and working to correct the muscle dysfunctions (a second year of physical therapy), she was searching for ways she could continue to live an active lifestyle. When she registered her daughter with LSI's program, she learned that they also taught lessons for adults. She became intrigued with the idea of using technical swimming as a safe way to exercise as she put her body back together. After taking the adult intermediate and then advanced courses for two years, she found that technical swimming combines the mind-body focus of yoga with cardio and resistance training. She learned that proper swimming technique improves posture and body alignment. She sees it as both challenging and calming. She's learning how to breathe properly and how to hold tension while staying relaxed. It allows her to apply what she learned in physical therapy and she feels she is harnessing an exercise that benefits her in so many ways. She can now see the truth in the LSI slogan, "Where swimming isn't just a sport, it's a necessity!"

In LSI Adult Clinic #2, students will work on lap swimming for Freestyle and Backstroke, and some will work on Breaststroke and Butterfly. By request, students can learn snorkeling, open-water swimming, and rescue swimming.

LIFESTYLE SWIMMING INSTRUCTION

LSI Advanced Adult Skills

Skill 1: Treads

Students warm up their bodies with treads across the pool and deck. Some will put their hands up, which we encourage. We look for relaxation. Treading should be quite effortless and relaxed at this level. They will continue working on relaxing legs and will learn not to work so hard in the water. The LSI method is *circle, touch, lean forward, chin over knees, round your back to bring hips up*. Pull water in front of you like giving yourself a hug. Feet go back, turn out, and do the Whip Kick with knees shoulder-width apart so feet don't go against the water.

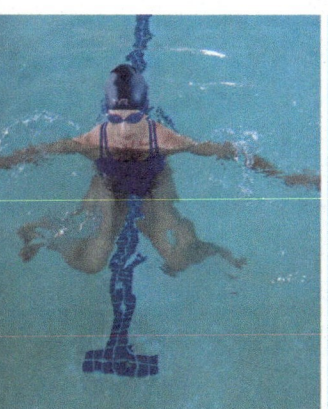

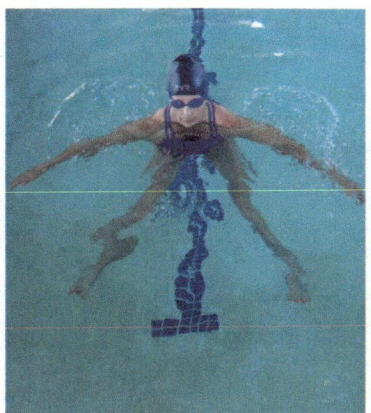

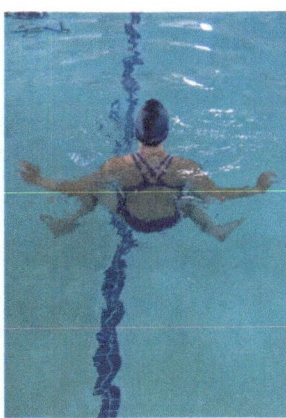

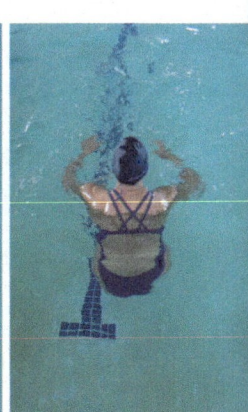

"IF YOU QUIT ONCE IT BECOMES A HABIT. NEVER QUIT!"

— MICHAEL JORDAN

Skill 2: Streamline

Students work on longer and faster Streamline, arms staying behind their ears and head in line with spine and breathing on second stroke, not first.

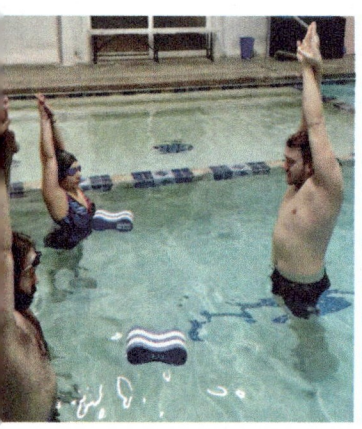

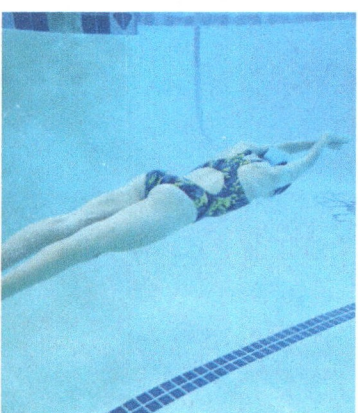

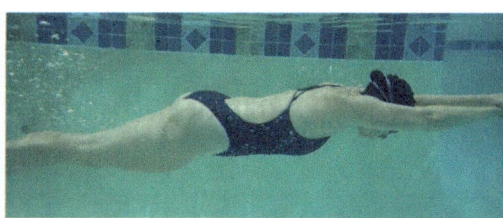

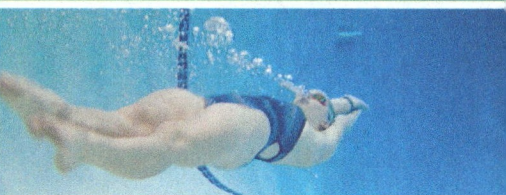

Skill 3: Lap Swimming for Freestyle

Students will try their best to swim a continual Freestyle for about five minutes while instructors correct them as needed.

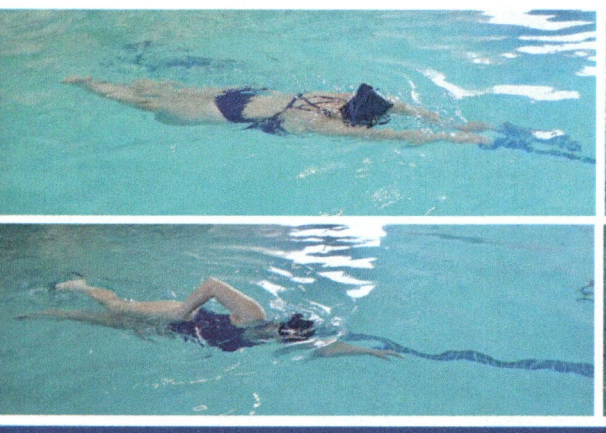

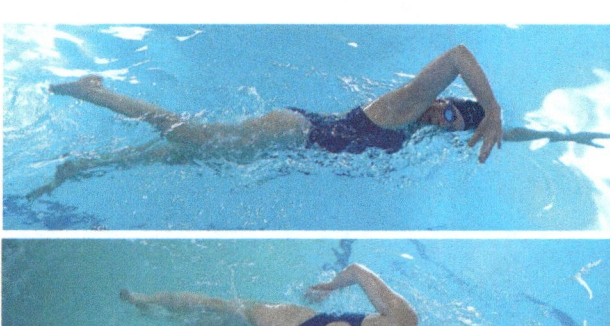

LIFESTYLE SWIMMING INSTRUCTION

Skill 4: Flip Turns

Once the students know how to do a flip turn, students will swim for five minutes nonstop, focusing on flip turns with proper form.

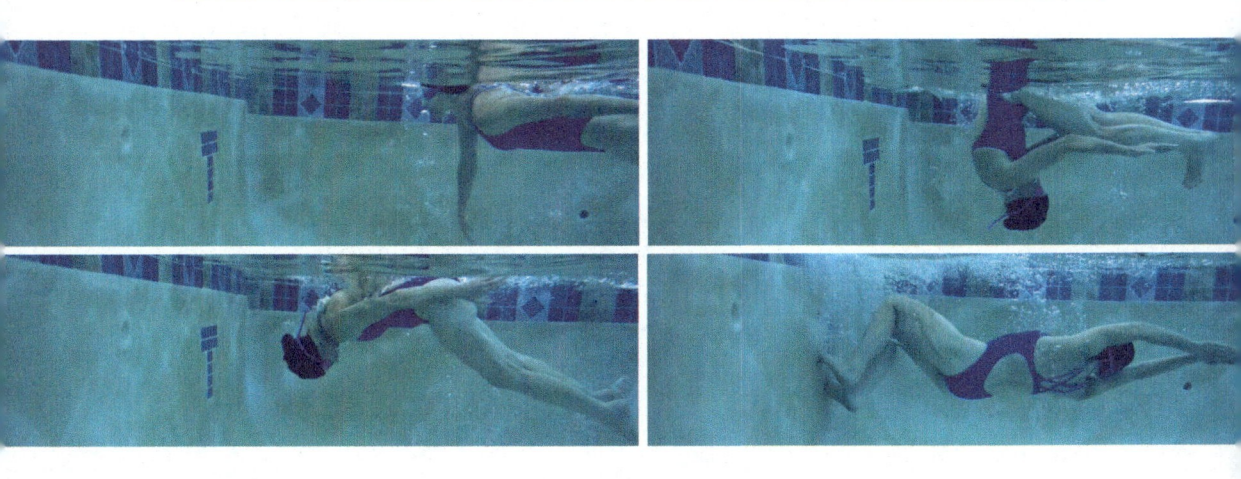

Skill 5: Lap Swimming for Backstroke

Students will get better with the Backstroke, working on correct timing for arms and flip turns on the wall to improve their swimming progress with more yardage.

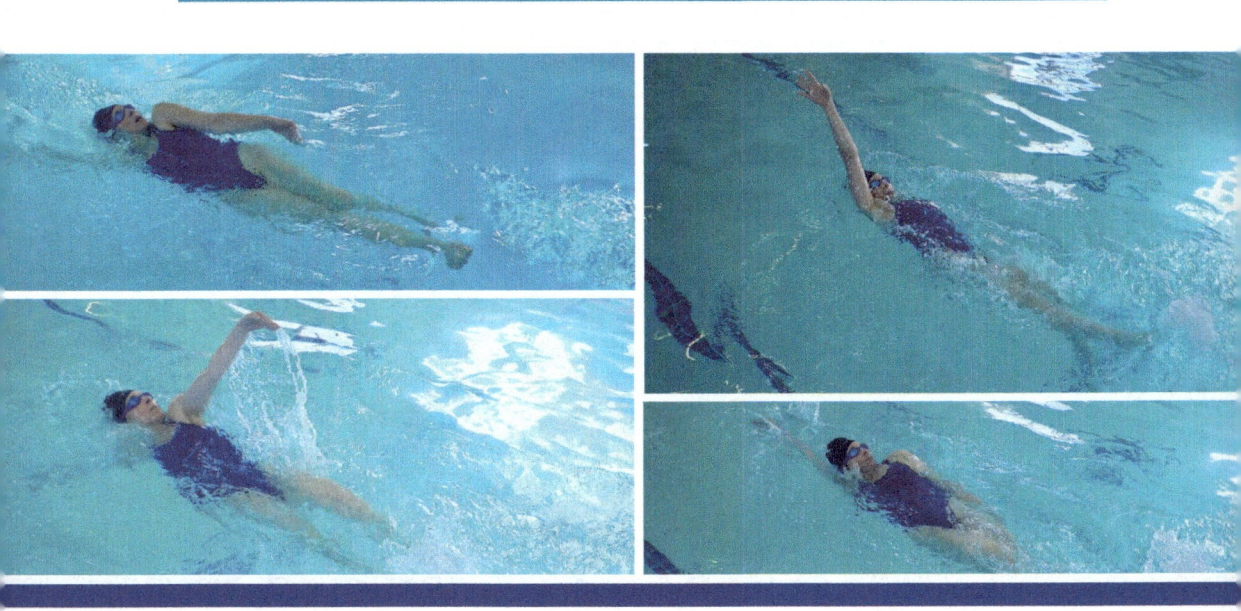

Skill 6: Introduce Drills and Improve Breaststroke

If it is the adult student's choice to keep learning more competitive strokes, we will teach them. Breaststroke is a favorite.

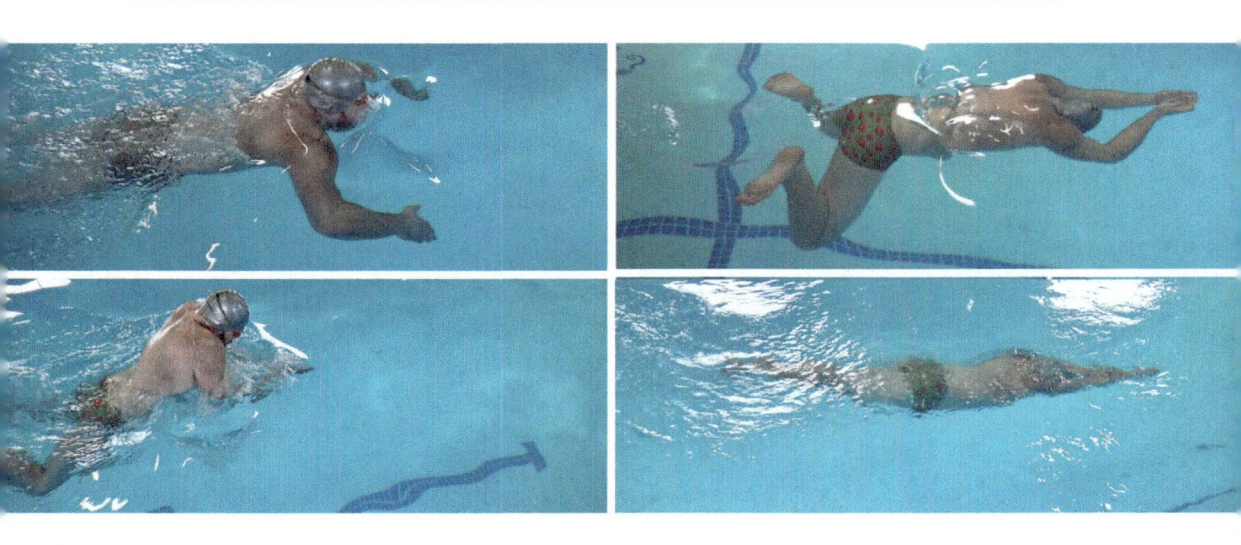

Skill 7: Introduce Drills and Improve Butterfly

Students do drills and learn how fluid their body needs to be in order to have the correct timing for their pull, kicks, and recovery for the Butterfly stroke.

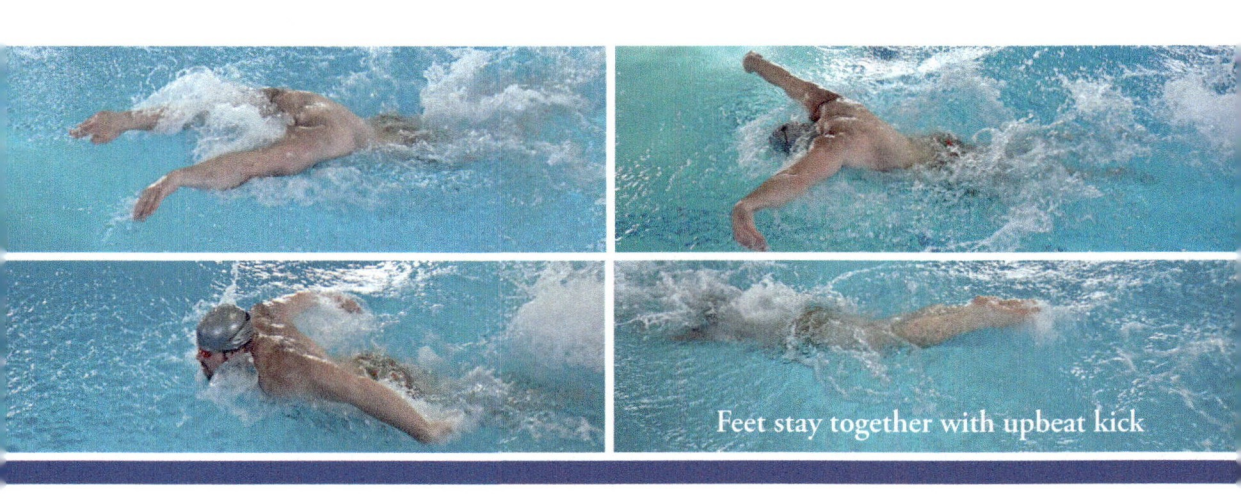

Feet stay together with upbeat kick

LIFESTYLE SWIMMING INSTRUCTION

Skill 8: Starting Dives

Students work on starting dives either for fun or competition.

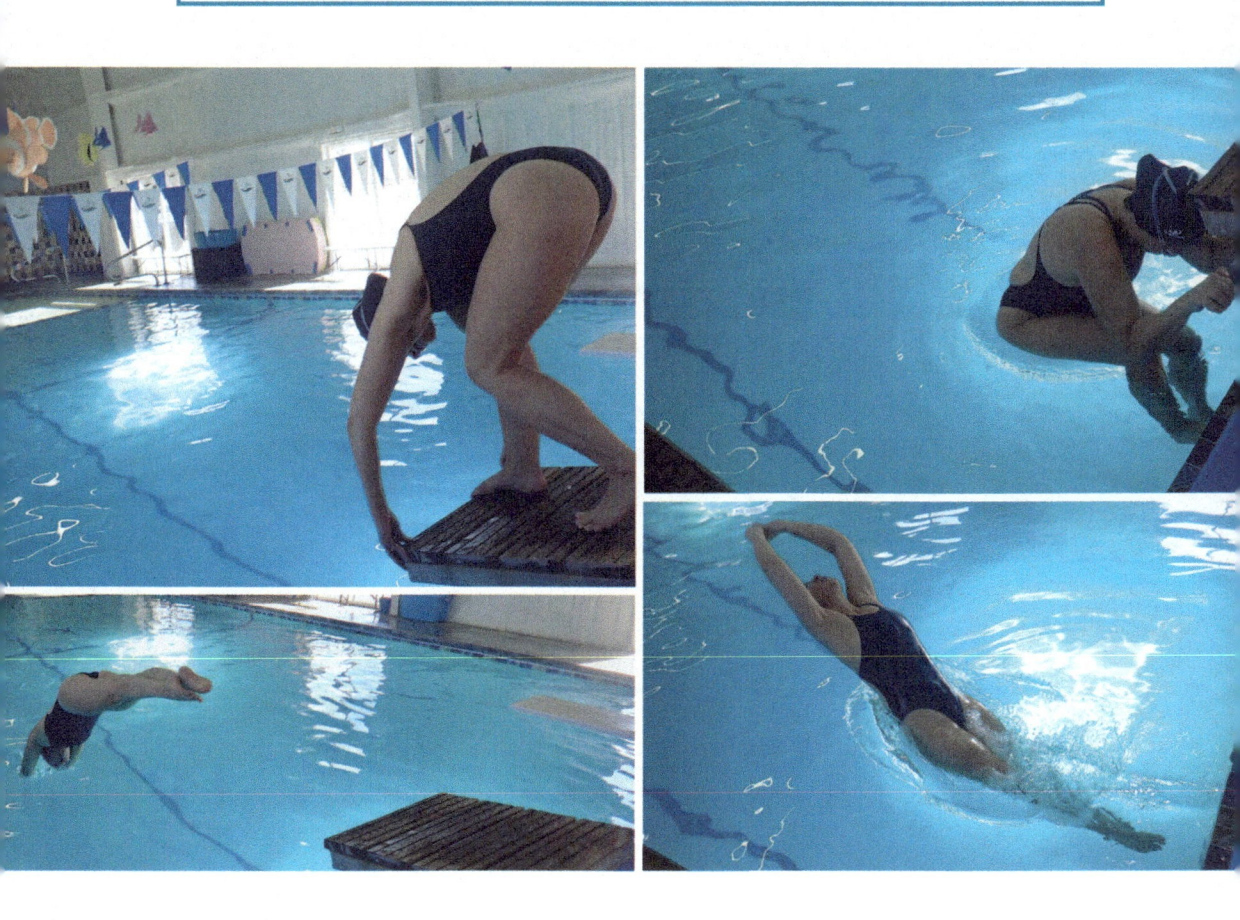

LSI CLINICS: ADULT INTERMEDIATE AND ADVANCED

ADULT INTERMEDIATE AND ADVANCED PARTING SHOTS

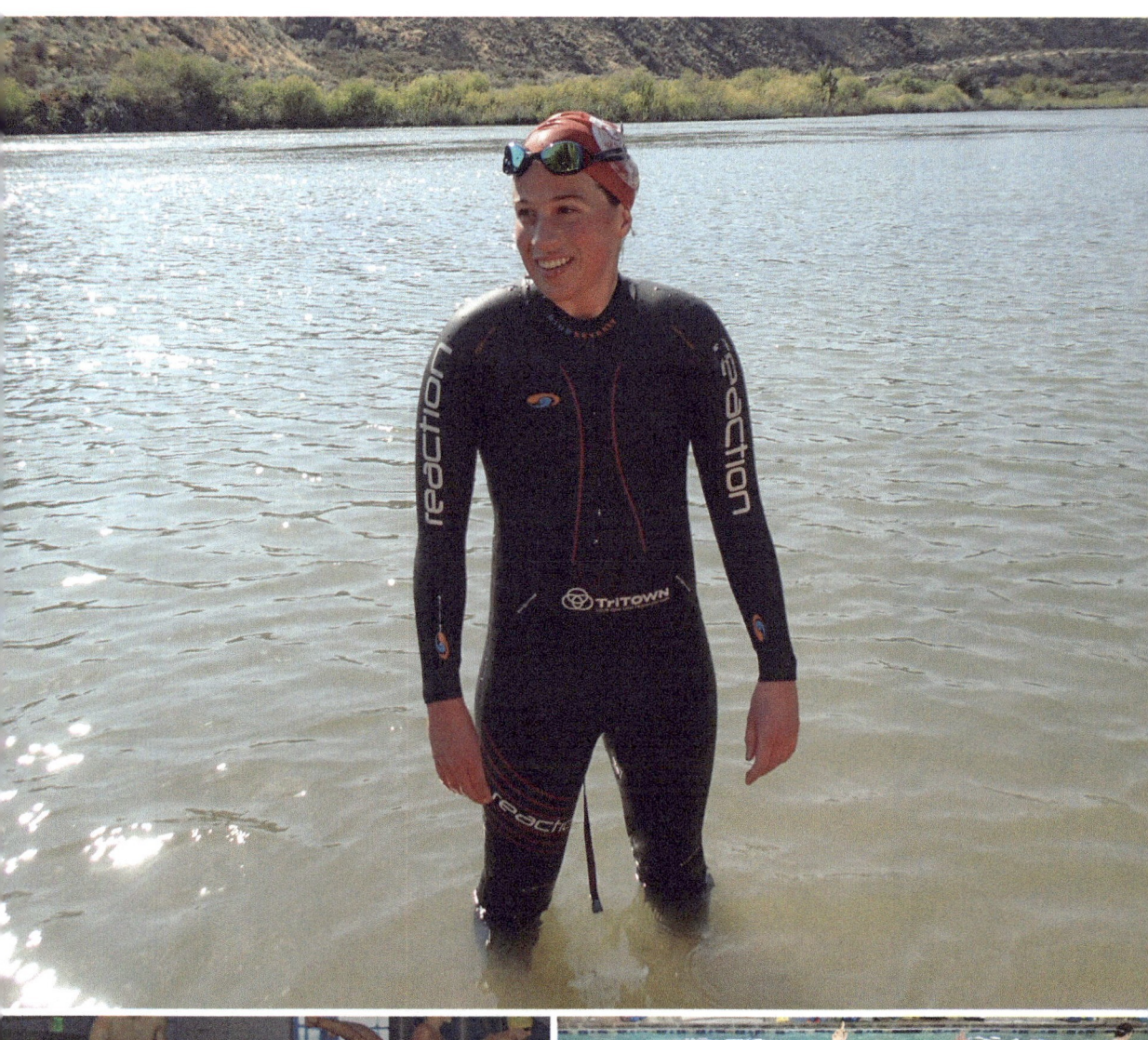

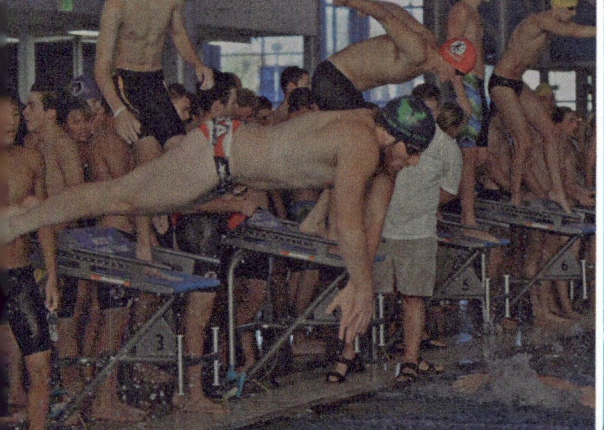

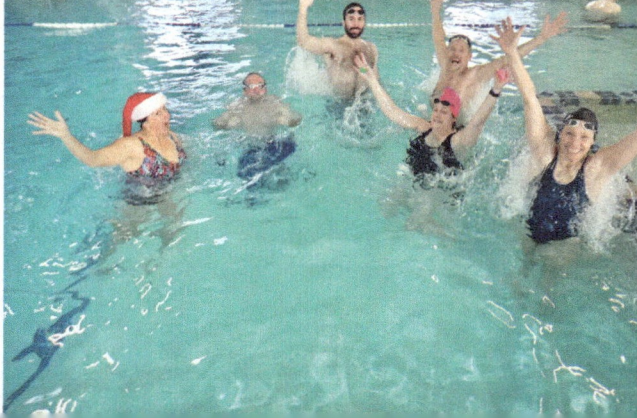

NOTES

CONCLUSION

Swimming is an important skill for everyone to learn. Having the ability to swim creates opportunities for fun and socialization, increases comfort and confidence both in and out of the water, and most importantly is a valuable safety skill. Everyone encounters water at some point in their life, and the ability to swim can be the difference between life and death.

Today the ability to swim is so common that those who can't may feel embarrassed about their inability or their fear of the water, keeping them from seeking the training they need to overcome this challenge. And for those who do know how to swim, many take it for granted. They can already swim, so why take lessons? Yet often people who already know how to swim are not swimming as well as they can or even should be. Their movements are inefficient, wasting energy and making swimming more difficult than it needs to be. They may not progress much in their skill despite taking lessons continuously.

Traditional swimming lessons are failing people. They don't focus on the way a body interacts with the water. But with a few changes to the way we approach lessons, anyone can learn to swim and swim well.

A good teaching method such as LSI's focuses on creating strong form from the beginning while building confidence in the water, learning to have fun, and most importantly, learning how the water and your body interact. Understanding how the water holds you and how you can move through it will improve your swimming at any level, allowing you to work with the water rather than fighting against it.

Swimming needs to be taught differently than it has been taught for so long. Lessons taught properly can help students overcome bad habits or fear of the water and can help students at any level progress and reach goals they never thought possible. With LSI's method, anyone can learn to swim confidently.

If you're a swimming instructor, compare your methods to the systematic approach outlined in this book. Are your students getting everything they need from you, in the right order? Are you building their confidence, teaching them to understand the properties of water, how it moves and works with them, and how to work with it instead of against it? Do you have a strong focus on form from the beginning? Are you able to correct errors in form or bad habits, and help even advanced students become better swimmers? You can do all of these things using LSI's approach to help your students get the most out of their instruction. I promise you, once you start, your students will never want to take lessons from anyone else.

If you are a frustrated parent who has continuously brought your children to swim lessons almost every month out of the year and they are still not swimming, there is a problem. They are not being taught. Always remember swimming isn't just about getting across the pool, but understanding *how* to get across the pool. Swimming is not just flopping around, it's a mindset and an ability to feel the water. Learn to be one with the water!

If you're a non-swimmer, a parent of a swim student, or a swim student yourself, take the initiative to do your research. Find an instructor who uses the LSI method so you can learn form and progress to higher levels of confidence. You can achieve your swimming goals!

ABOUT LIFESTYLE SWIMMING INSTRUCTION

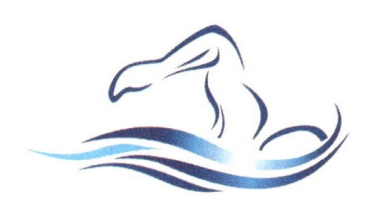

At LSI we create a safe, loving, and positive environment to give each student tools that teach bodies how to have the correct muscle memory so swimming is a process of growth and not a process of frustration. We motivate and fascinate students in fitness and learning to enrich their self-worth and self-esteem. We teach students in a loving way and give them the correct foundational skills so they will understand how to swim in any situation and never panic around the water. We believe that good swimmers need a solid foundation, so we teach you how to relax your body in a way that makes getting across the pool fluid and effortless. This takes time and practice. That is why LSI is taught year-round. Swimming doesn't just come naturally; it has to be taught correctly in order for you to swim correctly, like a fish, fluid and smooth. As Dory put it in *Finding Nemo*, "When life gets you down, just keep swimming!"

At LSI we want you to become comfortable both in and around water, improve your technique, set goals, and stay active! LSI students will walk away after every lesson knowing more than when they started. LSI teaches how the water works, safety skills, proper breathing, proper body position, and all the swim techniques necessary to progress and improve in all strokes. At the same time, students will also gain confidence in the water and get the exercise needed to live a healthy lifestyle.

The goal of LSI is to train instructors how to teach so people can learn to swim correctly. The instructors teach accurate technique to reduce body injury and improve water safety. They teach children that water is their friend but that they are not to enter any body of water without a parent. LSI instructors will educate families with backyard pools so drownings do not happen.

Our skills and lessons are designed to build on the previous level. Every student graduates from one level before going to the next level. When the student accomplishes all levels, they will graduate to be swim-team ready. This means when a graduate from LSI enters a swim team, they will be coachable, they will know how to differentiate what feels good and what doesn't, and they will be ready to increase their speed.

ACKNOWLEDGMENTS

I especially want to thank my family for being there for me, believing in me, and supporting me through this swimming journey.

I thank my parents for continuing to expose me to the water, whether it was pools or beaches, and putting up with me during all those years of screaming by the water.

First, I have to thank my mom. She was my first teacher and role model. Like most moms, she was the one who fed me, potty trained me, disciplined me, and in my case, taught me how to read and write. Our special bond extended past those beginning years before I started school because she was my kindergarten teacher. There was no slacking in her classroom. She gave me a gift from the beginning by teaching me to always give it my all and never put off something until tomorrow that can be done today! That is always in my mind and forever will be.

Thank you to my dad, who told me he always wanted me to write this book. I needed that inspiration!

Special thanks to my husband, Wade, who never thought he would have a second job as a "pool boy." Thank you for having the patience with my work in and out of the water, and especially for putting my pajamas in the dryer so they can be warm when I come in from the pool after working all day! I love that you love me!

Special thanks to God for all of his goodness and for giving us three blessings from above: Brittany, Ryan, and Jay. They are the reason I started Lifestyle Swimming Instruction, LLC.

Thank you to those three blessings, Brittany, Ryan, and Jay, for swimming, competing, and working, sometimes all in the same day; for your hard work and great work ethic with all ages of people; and for your wonderful conversations and insights into what you believed swimming should and shouldn't be. I will always cherish our early morning snuggles and late-night conversations, laughs, and tears over hot specialty drinks we found on Pinterest!

Thank you to all past and present instructors who work or have worked hard and are or were an asset to LSI! I love how some of you come back and teach when you have breaks from school and life in general. I love to see it come full circle when you get married and have kids and see your little ones in our LSI swim lessons.

Thanks to my friends and LSI families who helped mold my swimming instructional career and encouraged me to write this book. Thank you for your consistency in bringing your children to swim lessons, session after session, year after year, and for understanding that "Swimming is not just a sport, it's a necessity!" Some families have turned into friends, and I am so grateful to have you all in my life. I would list you all, but there are so many and you all know who you are.

I am so grateful for my publisher, Maryanna, for going to the same convention I went to and approaching me, asking me what I did. That day was the beginning of a dream I only hoped would come true. Thank you for taking me in, having patience with my swim schedule, and believing in me and LSI. You gave me a desire to put things into words and opened the door to make this possible.

Thank you to Aloha Publishing team member Heather for your patience with rough draft after rough draft, picture after picture, and redo after redo, not to mention flash drives that were blank! Thank you for coming to a clinic so you could see first-hand how things work here at LSI.

ACKNOWLEDGMENTS

Thank you, Nancy, my bookkeeper, for being my angel like no other. You taught me more than you could possibly know how to run things in and out of the pool. Your positive life approach and always saying you are "just ducky" gets me through so many days. I cannot express enough how grateful my family and I are for you to have come into our lives. Thank you too, Louanne, for coming into my life. I am so glad you came here to learn to swim and got Nancy to come. Life just wouldn't be the same without you two in our lives. I also love the fact that I am in your mind when you swim during your retirement years!

Thank you to all my active models for the photo shoots to make this book become a reality: Ryan, Lillian, Amy, Vivianne, Charli, Jaqueline, Evelyn, and all others who helped take the pictures or pose in some way. I am so grateful for you all taking the time out of your days!

A special thanks to my first coach, Steve, who taught me so much about the swimming world and opened my eyes to a world I never knew about. You planted the seed of swimming knowledge that put me on a crazy life journey I never imagined. Thank you for pushing me to my limits, even when Robyn and I thought you were torturing us.

A special thanks to Coach Jonathan, who was the coach I took my three children to on a vacation so they could do swim practices while being away. He was the exact coach I dreamed for them to have. Thank you for keeping a connection with me, always answering my emails or phone calls, and being a great mentor, not to mention the best coach I have ever witnessed!

And thank you to all of our students who come in and tell us they love us, want to have hot chocolate with us, give us hugs, and learn to say, "I will try!"

NOTES

ABOUT THE AUTHOR

Susanne told her parents when she was in second grade, "I was born to make noise!"

She sees the world differently. She grew up in a non-swimming world, which intrigued and challenged her to learn how to swim. She went to many places to help her achieve this goal, but it ended up being an educational process that led to her quest to find the right way to teach swimming.

Susanne was born in Burbank, Illinois. Her family moved to Downers Grove, Illinois, when she was in first grade. During her ninth-grade year, she moved to Los Alamos, New Mexico. After meeting her husband there and going to college in Albuquerque, they moved to Boise, Idaho, where they have raised three wonderful children who all entered the competitive swimming world and worked teaching swimming lessons for their family-owned and operated business.

Susanne worked with children from the time she was a young girl, helping her mom in her classroom. After taking many swim classes, she was told she should teach swimming. She became obsessed with learning the correct way of swimming from the start and that intrigued her to dig deep and learn the sport from the inside out. She taught swimming at the YMCA for several years and designed her own lesson plans. On the days she worked, she juggled taking her children to school and back to the YMCA after school for swim team practices.

LIFESTYLE SWIMMING INSTRUCTION

She assisted in coaching a high school swim team one season and then realized she loved the competition side as well as the learning side. She swam, trained, and learned from collegiate and national-level swimmers by helping them with clinics and studying the hows and whys of the swimming community. She went out on her own when a past swim instructor retired and wanted her to take her clientele.

Susanne founded Lifestyle Swimming Instruction in 2005 to offer her community an alternative to "ordinary" swim lessons. Susanne is a firm believer in education and understanding before students do anything in the water. She believes that if her students understand the whys and hows, the muscle memory in the mind and body will connect.

Susanne has taught swimming for over 20 years. She specializes in teaching all ages, helping students overcome aquaphobia and learn safety and competitive swimming. Her educational background was elementary education until she saw a need for better instruction in the swimming world. She is excited to extend this knowledge to others by offering this proven method of teaching.

Susanne loves spending time with family and friends. Outside of the pool, she enjoys a good cup of hot chocolate made from scratch, kitchen creations for a good home-cooked meal, and interior designing. She enjoys mountain biking, skiing, snowmobiling, hiking, camping, visiting family, and traveling.

CONNECT WITH LSI

Susanne would like to share her revolutionary swimming method by training instructors and educating parents, students, and communities around the world. If you are interested in learning or teaching swimming the LSI way, connect with Susanne:

Facebook: Lifestyle Swimming Instruction, LLC
Instagram: @LSIswim
Website: LSIswim.com
Email: info@LSIswim.com

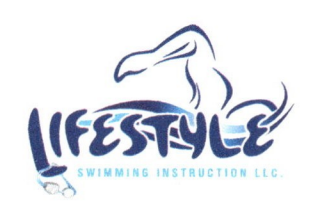

Made in the USA
Columbia, SC
28 November 2022